The
GREENING
of
MEDICINE

Patrick Pietroni

FRGCP MRCP DCH

LONDON
VICTOR GOLLANCZ LTD
1991

First published in Great Britain 1990
by Victor Gollancz Ltd
14 Henrietta Street, London WC2E 8QJ

First published in Gollancz Paperbacks 1991

ISBN 0 575 05043 8

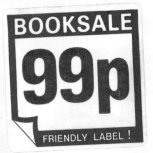

Photoset by Rowland Phototypesetting Ltd,
Bury St Edmunds, Suffolk
Printed in Great Britain by
Guernsey Press Co. Ltd, Guernsey, Channel Isles

Dr Patrick C Pietroni, FRCGP, MRCP, DCH, is Senior Lecturer in General Practice at St Mary's Hospital Medical School, London, past Chairman of the British Holistic Medical Association, and a Jungian analyst. He is also principal partner in the Marylebone Health Centre, set up in 1986, which aims 'to explore and evaluate ways in which primary health care can be delivered to a deprived area in addition to the General Practice component. The approaches include an holistic component comprising an educational self help model with a complementary medical model'. As a result of this experiment the Marylebone Centre Trust was founded in 1988 to expand the work of the Marylebone Health Centre.

Dr Pietroni is married with three children and lives in North London.

By the same author

HOLISTIC LIVING

To George Engel

Contents

Foreword

The changes taking place within our society during the latter part of this century have provided challenges in many different aspects of our lives. Rising interest in the preservation of our environment has grown out of concerns ranging from the pollution of the North Sea to the purity of our drinking water. Medicine has always involved itself with improving the quality of life and it is appropriate that many of these changes to which we are now subject are having an impact on the way medicine is practised. Indeed, it is important that health-care practitioners of all kinds continue to adapt to the different needs of the times.

In Britain and the developed world the diseases of the nineteenth century have largely been eradicated through improvements in both social and medical practice. We have as yet to address successfully the epidemics of the twentieth century. During my presidency of the BMA I suggested medicine might re-explore some of the more traditional approaches that have been neglected by orthodox science. In the intervening eight years, several initiatives by the Royal Society of Medicine, the British Medical Association and the Royal College of General Practitioners have resulted in a dialogue from which new and exciting developments continue to occur.

Some of these developments are described in detail within this book. Dr Pietroni, whose own contribution in this area has been enormous, has helped to map out both these developments, and others, that owe a great deal to the courage, ingenuity and creativity of many practitioners both within and outside the traditional practice of medicine.

Acknowledgements

To write a book of this kind which attempts to bring together many disciplines and several languages of health care inevitably means that most of the material is not original. To acknowledge every source would prove an enormous task, yet I am aware that without the inspiration and guidance from many colleagues, the task would have been impossible. Similarly, in the last few years I have been fortunate to receive generous financial support from several sources to enable me to explore the concepts in a very practical manner. In particular I would like to thank members of the Wates Foundation who have been personally supportive as well as financially generous. Sir Maurice Laing has over the years of our acquaintance, kept a watchful and guiding eye over the work and ensured that its progress retains a level of professionalism that it might otherwise have lacked. Lord Kindersley has offered advice that enabled the political dimension of the work to be acknowledged and addressed.

I am particularly grateful to Sir James Watt and Sir David Innes-Williams for reading the draft and proffering both supportive and constructive criticisms. Dick Thompson helped me to rethink the first section and added to the weight of the historical argument. Ann Kilkoyne's research on inter-professional issues formed the basis of the final section of Chapter 7, and Mark Pietroni was particularly helpful in rewriting the chapter on cancer.

Special thanks are owed to Christopher Hamel-Cooke, whose vision and unceasing efforts have made possible the development of the Crypt at St Marylebone Church.

To have an opportunity to explore new ideas in the context of a busy NHS general practice is rare indeed and without the support of my colleagues at the Marylebone Health Centre and Marylebone Centre Trust, little of what is in this book would have seen the light of day. They have had to tolerate a degree of change and uncertainty whilst at the same time providing a structure that allowed for these ideas to take root. They have also had to tolerate the 'messiness' that is inevitable in a venture of this kind. Ros Tennyson, Derek Chase and Peter Davies have not only held my hand but added their own particular expertise to the shaping of this experiment.

I am indebted to Mary Toase who both proof-read and checked the references, a valuable if thankless task.

During the gestation and writing of this book, I have been supported and more importantly been understood by Moira Jenkins who has typed several drafts and offered her own perceptive comments to each one. Finally, to live what one believes is never easy, and certainly I would plead guilty to many failures. However, without my wife Marilyn's influence these failures would have ensured that this book could not have been written.

I would like also to thank the following for permission to reproduce tables and diagrams: American Psychiatric Association for Figures 2 and 3, taken from *The American Journal of Psychiatry*, 137:5, May 1980, p. 537, article by G. C. Engel; Basil Blackwell Ltd for Figures 11 and 12, taken from *The Captured Womb* by Ann Oakley, 1984; Edward Arnold (Publishers) Ltd for Figure 13 and Table 8, taken from *The Management of Terminal Malignant Disease* by Dame Cicely Saunders, 1984; Hodder & Stoughton Ltd (Coronet Books) for Tables 14 and 15, taken from *The Handbook of Complementary Medicine* by Stephen Fulder; Open University Press for Figures 8 and 9, taken from *The Woman in the Body* by Emily Martin, 1989; Prometheus Books, New York, for Figure 14, taken from *The Faith Healers* by James Randi, 1987; Routledge & Kegan Paul Ltd for Figure 10, taken from *A Dictionary of Symbols* by J. E. Carlot, 1962, and Table 2, taken from *The Awakening Earth* by Peter Russell, 1982; Thames and Hudson Ltd for Figure 7, taken from *An Illustrated Encyclopaedia of Traditional Symbols* by J. C. Cooper, 1978; William Collins Sons & Co. Ltd (Fontana) for Figure 1, taken from *The Coming of the Greens* by Jonathon Porritt.

Introduction

The life of a junior hospital doctor in a London teaching hospital in the Sixties was full of paradoxes. One night I was helping a now famous heart surgeon perform an 'emergency' mechanical heart transplant on the floor, in a hospital ward, behind closed curtains, to the consternation of a silent audience of wide-awake patients, and the next night, with equal drama and the same amount of adrenalin flowing through my veins, I was listening to the Beatles to the delight of a highly vocal audience. Both events were the forerunners of changes to come within medicine and society. The first, an example of the 'hero in medicine' which laid the ground-work for the technological advances of live transplants, in-vitro fertilisation, genetic engineering and human embryo research. The second, an example of another form of breakthrough – that of music, ideas and feelings that were to 'unite the world' around a pop group and Bob Geldof, twenty-five years later.

Medical progress in the second half of this century has largely ignored this second breakthrough and one could say it has developed in isolation of the world of ideas and feelings. That this state of affairs can no longer continue has been clear for some time. The bedrock on which much of modern medical practice is based is too narrow to encompass the needs and demands that are now required of it. The intellectual framework underpinning the curricula of most Western medical schools has not incorporated the developing world of ideas and feelings into their structure. The world has moved on and medicine is in danger of being left behind. Medical students are still taught that medicine is, by and large, about the body and its functions; that the body is made up of bits and pieces which are studied as separate and distinct entities. They are still taught about the mind as a separate entity from the body. They are still taught that treatment comes either in the form of a prescription or a surgical operation. They receive little or no training in communication skills and leave medical school with an understanding of disease but no knowledge of health. This impoverished and narrow education is a far cry from the humanist tradition from which the study of medicine arose – one which was steeped in the world of ideas and feelings. As a nursing sister working at St. Christopher's Hospice said – 'Feelings are facts in this place'.

Feelings must indeed again become facts within the discipline of medicine. For as we struggle to resolve the problems of the undoubted success of Western social and scientific progress, we find that our old and trusted methods no longer provide us with the solutions; indeed they appear to compound the problems. Progress has to take place not only in the world of technology but in the world of ideas and feelings. New forms of technology will no doubt follow once the new ideas have taken root – that is the way of man's progress. The form these new ideas will take is as yet uncertain but for the moment they appear best described by the epithet 'Green'. Like all new movements a certain amount of scepticism is appropriate. However, what I have tried to indicate in this book is that Green ideas are not new; they were always there, ready to be discovered and used by man when the need arose. The need has now arisen and we see the application of many of these ideas in our social life. Medicine cannot and must not be left behind – it is too central to the life of the nation and to the daily experience of millions of people.

In Part One of the book I try to outline in a condensed form some of the historical origins of Green ideas with special relevance to medical practice. This section can be bypassed and possibly more profitably read last. Part Two outlines the current crisis – for crisis it is that medicine is facing. This is not another anti-doctor book, for my hope is to help steer medicine back to its true path, the one trodden by Hippocrates, Asclepiades, Paracelsus, Osler, Medawar and, most recently, Oliver Sacks. If feelings are to become facts in this renaissance in medicine, then certainly some of the facts in this section will arouse feelings. This cannot be avoided – medicine needs to rekindle its passion and radical edge for it to effect the changes required of it. Part Three includes some, but by no means all, of the examples of the greening process that have already taken root within medical practice. Isolated examples some may be but each in its own right deserves recognition for breakthroughs as important as the heart transplants of main-stream medicine. It is on these seeds and others like them that the future healthy growth of medicine depends.

PART I

Setting the Scene

1

New Gods – Old Worlds

The quiet revolution

There is a revolution coming. It will not be like revolutions of the past. It will originate in the individual and with culture and it will change the political structure only as its final act. It will not require violence to succeed and it cannot be successfully resisted with violence. It is now spreading with amazing rapidity and already our laws, institutions and social structure are changing in consequence. It promises a higher reason, a more humane community and a new and liberated individual. Its ultimate creation will be a new and enduring wholeness and beauty – a renewed relationship of man to himself, to other men, to society, to nature and to the land.

Charles Reich, *The Greening of America*[1]

On re-reading *The Greening of America*, twenty years after its publication in 1970, it is easy to adopt a somewhat lofty and dismissive attitude towards some of Reich's more idealistic global prophecies.

Writing, as he was, during a period of American history when the peace movement drew fire from supporters of the Vietnam War and 'flower children' ran the gauntlet with the National Guard, it is perhaps understandable that his vision of Utopia should have reflected his sense of hope for the future more accurately than his ability to predict its outcome.

As we sit glued to our television sets, witnessing the tearing down of the Berlin Wall and the emergent democracies of Eastern Europe demanding the right to freedom and a better quality of life, on reflection, perhaps Reich was right. Revolutions can originate in the individual and with culture, and they can change political structures after all.

The mark of great innovative thinkers is that they not only

advance new ideas, but are also prepared to be proved wrong. The 'Green Revolution' of the past two decades owes its success not simply to the hard-fought battles of environmentalists, but to the open-mindedness of debate across a wide spectrum of political, social and environmental concern.

Reich pointed the way forward in a clear and uncompromising manner because he recognised the depth of the crisis then present in American society – corruption, social disorder, poverty, inequality, uncontrolled technology, the destruction of the environment, the artificiality of work and culture, the absence of community and the loss of self. His own solution focused upon the need for a new consciousness in which self-awareness, genuineness, authenticity and social organisation filter through to replace the negative features of a society seemingly bent on its own destruction.

No doubt because he was writing at the end of the Sixties, many of his ideas were labelled 'cranky' by critics who associated 'Green ideas' with the narcissistic self-absorption of a 'lost' generation. The durability of these ideas over the past twenty years, however, proves that Reich was correct in his assertion that the revolution was coming, though not, perhaps, as quickly as he might have wished, nor so evidently in the America for which he held out such high hopes.

It is important to distinguish between words like 'Green' and phrases like 'the Green Revolution'. Green ideas have been variously connected with concerns ranging from feminism, animal rights and environmentalism to the peace movement and consumerism. Originally, the Green Revolution was a phrase used to describe new high-yield wheat strains that had been developed in Mexico and were subsequently exported to India to help solve the sub-continent's chronic food shortages.

In *The Coming of the Greens* (1988), Jonathon Porritt acknowledges that 'Green' tends to mean different things to different people. He differentiates between the 'light Greens', or environmentalists, and the 'dark Greens', or radicalists.[2] Clearly concern for the environment is central to all Green thinking. Petitioning for the cessation of a motorway or the preservation of a wild-life sanctuary are quintessential Green issues. Concern over the pollution of rivers or the dumping of nuclear waste is now at the forefront of public debate and is no longer merely a fringe or counter-culture activity.

Figure 1 The ideology and structure of modern environmentalism

Eco-centrism		*Techno-centrism*	
Gaianism belief in the rights of nature and of the essential co-evolution of humans and natural phenomena	*Communalism* belief in the co-operation capabilities of societies to be collectively self-reliant using 'appropriate' science and technology	*Accommodation* faith in the adaptability of institutions and mechanisms of assessment and decision-making to accommodate to environmental demands	*Optimism* faith in the application of science, market forces and managerial ingenuity
redistribution of power towards a decentralized, federal political economy based on the interlinkage of environmental and social justice	→	← maintenance of the status quo in existing structures of government power	

Source: T. O'Riordan Discussion Paper OECD 1983.

Even amongst environmentalists, however, major divisions exist over appropriate approaches to these problems. Tom O'Riordan provides a helpful analysis of the modern environmentalism movement.

While the radical Greens show concern for how we relate to our environment, they stress equally the importance of how we relate to each other and to other species. Ultimately, Green issues become political and social issues, because at every level they impinge upon the quality of our lives and upon the environments in which we live.

To be a Green now carries the connotation of political involvement. In 1984, Fritjof Capra and Charlene Spretnak argued that the emergence of Green politics 'is an ecological, holistic and feminist movement that transcends the old political framework of left versus right. It emphasises the interconnectedness and interdependence of all phenomena, as well as the embeddedness of individuals and societies in the cyclical process of nature. It addresses the unjust and destructive dynamics of the patriarchy. It calls for social responsibility and a sound, sustainable economic system, one that is ecological, decentralised, equitable and compromised of flexible institutions, one in which people have significant control over their lives'.[3]

By the late 1980s, the Green movement within Europe was witnessing a major expansion in its popularity. Beginning with a distinct political party in Germany, the movement gained credibility by forming loose coalitions with existing political parties. As the impact of its appeal began to be felt across national frontiers, governments in neighbouring countries started to adopt 'Green issues' as if they had always been central to their political philosophies. In Britain, Margaret Thatcher claimed legitimacy for 'Green politics' by claiming that 'we are all environmentalists now'.

A movement capable of producing the kind of changes in political thinking that we have witnessed over the past few years undoubtedly influences the major institutions and corporate bodies whose power extends deep within the societies in which we live. As the commercial giants clamour to adopt the Green image, how long, we ask ourselves, will it be before the major professions of law, medicine and religion follow suit?

It is curious that within the profession of medicine little credence is given to the significance to the contributions provided by public health and epidemiology. Despite the fact that the dramatic fall in death rates in the Western world since the latter part of the nineteenth century can be ascribed to environmental improvements such as water purification and sewage disposal, such contributions are rarely accredited with having stimulated medical advance.

Similarly, nutrition, which at various times gains popularity with doctors in the prevention and management of ill-health, rates low on the list of medical specialisms. Now that Green awareness is spreading throughout the multimillion pound health-food and fitness industries, the medical profession is being forced by the public to respond more sensitively to questions concerning personal health management.

In much the same way that Reich's quiet revolution espouses the principles of harmony, balance, the interconnectedness of natural phenomena and the search for inner awareness, so too will the revolution in twenty-first century medicine. The growth of the 'consciousness industry' has already had a considerable influence upon personal health care, popularised by such books as *Anatomy of an Illness,*[4] *Love, Medicine and Miracles,*[5] and *You Can Fight for Your Life.*[6] All suggest that the possibility of effecting change in one's state of well-being derives from altering one's consciousness of self and one's relationship with the environment.

However, before medicine, with its empirical focus upon diagnosing and curing dis-ease, is in a position to embrace Green concepts, a fundamental shift of attitude has yet to occur. The sole dependence upon science and the rational-scientific approach to knowledge is deeply engrained within our culture. Notions of progress and civilisation rest firmly upon such foundations. The successes of modern medicine appear writ in tablets of stone.

It is to these issues that we now turn.

The ascent of reason

There is not any haunt of prophecy,
Nor any old chimera of the grave,
Neither the golden underground, nor isle
Melodious, where spirits got them home,
Nor visionary youth, nor cloudy palm
Remote on heaven's hill, that has endured
As April's green endures; or will endure
                                    Wallace Stevens

It is ironic that the contemporary use of the word 'Green', despite its positive emphasis on the need for global awareness, should, in fact, have derived from a reaction to the mis-use of nature. For five hundred years man's obsession with taming the forces of nature has gone hand-in-glove with his aspiration to make science the arbiter of all known things.

From the moment that the early navigators discovered the eastern seaboard of the Americas, fear of the unknown gave way to mathematical calculation and rational planning. Secure in the knowledge that they would not topple over the edge of the world, the stage was set for mercantile expansion and the exploitation of the New World. Material wealth was to become the principle upon which power could be wielded and social status and privilege secured. Understandably, little thought was given to the human or environmental consequences of such expansion.

The explosion of Reason during the Renaissance heralded a major shift in thinking about the relationship between God and

Man. By the time of Copernicus's death in 1543, his 'Revolution of
the Celestial Bodies' was already fuelling the fires of debate
initiated by Lutheran reformism. New thinking was dangerous,
even heretical. To suggest that the earth revolved around the sun
not only weakened the authority of the Church but suggested that
knowledge was attainable through reasoned thought as distinct
from ecclesiastical teaching or divine revelation.

As Galileo was establishing the proof of the Copernican hypothesis, Descartes was laying the foundations for rational scientific
enquiry. His famous dictum 'I think, therefore I am', was particularly significant in that he was confirming the march of Reason
through territory traditionally dominated by ecclesiastical authority. Man was beginning to free himself from the dogma of the
Church and preparing the ground for a new kind of authority –
rational science.

By the time of the publication of Newton's *Principia* in 1687,
few vestiges of the 'old world' remained. The 'celestial orbs'
moved through space in perfect, defined motion. Life was no
longer 'nasty, brutish and short', as Hobbes had described it sixty
years earlier. Descartes' philosophical dualism had separated the
physical from the metaphysical and hence mind from body and
Man from God. In his search for a unified philosophy whereby
men would become 'masters and possessors of nature', Descartes
broke with the imprecise and occult traditions of mediaeval
science to pursue a universally applicable method of establishing
verifiable knowledge. It was not that he sought to reject
metaphysics or the use of Pure Reason, rather that he doubted the
veracity of their employment. Better to start from a position of
scepticism, he argued, and to deduce answers from logical formu-
lae, than to assume the Mind as being capable of independently
verifying universal truths.

Whether or not Descartes is responsible for the mistakes that
science has made in respect of Man and Nature over the past three
hundred years cannot obscure the fact that it was his systematic
method that gave rise to the mechanistic, reductionist and dual-
istic concepts that have since become the hallmarks of rational-
scientific enquiry. 'I consider the human body as a machine,' he
wrote. 'My thought compares a sick man and an ill-made clock
with my ideas of a healthy man and a well-made clock. I say that
you consider these functions occur naturally in this machine solely
by the dispositions of its organs not less than the movement of a

clock.' Just as Hobbes learned from Galileo's reconstructions of complex physical problems that even moral issues could be broken down to their constituent parts and then rebuilt to sub-stantiate their logical meaning, so too did Descartes in his analysis of the relationship between mind and body. There is always a need, he wrote, 'to divide each of the difficulties into as many parts as possible and as might be necessary for its adequate solution.[7]

From Copernicus to Galileo and Descartes to Newton, the story of the rational pursuit of knowledge parallels the imposition of natural law over religion. The more confident that Man became about his ability to predict and control nature, the less he cared about the consequences of his actions. It was not that God was at fault for nature's imperfections, rather that since Man had ac-quired Reason, he was now better armed to confront nature directly.

Throughout the seventeenth and eighteenth centuries the growth of Reason was clearly regarded as being pivotal to scientific progress and commercial expansion. However, as rational idealist and empiricist thinkers fought each other for the higher intellec-tual and moral ground, a bifurcation in the expression – and verification – of new ideas began to take effect within Europe. Whereas idealist thinking, from Plato to Kant, emphasised the primacy of mind over matter and form over content in the rational pursuit of knowledge, empiricists chose to rely upon experience and observation rather than pure reason, remaining sceptical of all attempts to provide general theoretical explanations or universal truths. Materialists, on the other hand, simply believed that all facts were causally dependent upon physical processes or were ultimately reducible to them.

While rationalism continued to flourish in continental Europe, empiricism established a firm hold in Britain. Hume's famous doctrine that all significant statements can be divided between those which concern matters of fact (experience, observation) and relations between ideas (incapable of proof), was to have a long-lasting effect upon the relationship between science and metaphysics and between Man and Nature.

By the mid-nineteenth century, the empirical sciences were giving rise to speculation that even the most fundamental ques-tions relating to the origin of species could be answered. Sup-ported by a better educated and secular public, Lamarck and

Darwin propounded theories of evolution that challenged traditional religious views on The Creation. Although the notion of inevitability bore greater resemblance to European idealist theories of universal causation than to the hard-and-fast reductionism of nineteenth-century scientific theory, the careful, analytic procedure for the presentation of facts to bear out the argument certainly did not.

Whilst the biological and physical sciences were making their reputations on the basis of their ability to explain the complexities of natural phenomena, scientific medicine was establishing its claim to improvements in the quality of ordinary people's lives. Riding on the back of successes in the control of the major infectious diseases, the profession of medicine consolidated its position as the rightful authority over matters of health and welfare.

In the space of three hundred years, the ascent of Reason had given rise to distinctly separate models of rational enquiry. Whereas the rational-idealist tradition within Europe had felt able to reconcile universal or holistic theories with deductive principles of scientific methodology, the Cartesian and empiricist traditions continued to reject such theories, preferring instead the reductionist approach whereby universals could only derive from the elucidation of particular elements.

Despite the enormous advances in knowledge made during the nineteenth and early twentieth centuries, the problem that empirical science was beginning to face was that progress was often bought at the expense of Nature. As physicists recognised the folly of separating scientific enquiry from responsibility in the production of nuclear weapons, so too did biologists in the creation of chemical warfare. In medicine, scientific progress in genetic manipulation, transplant surgery and embryo research has led to major ethical questions which for the most part doctors have found themselves ill-prepared to address. As governments and corporate giants have utilised science in the cause of economic and commercial expansion, so the earth's natural resources have been systematically depleted.

The absence of accountability in science has gone hand-in-glove with the wholesale exploitation of Man and Nature. Now, as we reach the end of the twentieth century, we appear set to reap the whirlwind. And yet, as we stare global disaster in the face, a groundswell of reaction is emerging which prefaces a movement away from reductionist science, towards a more ecologically sound approach to knowledge and, thereby, to Nature.

What is now required is not a wholesale rejection of reductionistic science or indeed a move away from rational thought. The call to return to 'natural laws' needs to be viewed with suspicion and concern – for the call is often fuelled by fear and nostalgia of a romanticised view of nature. The task is far more difficult than is often acknowledged by many 'new age' writers. We require all the insights and truths that the age of Reason has brought us. However, using the image of a 'cosmic relay race', the torch of progress that has for so long been carried by the descendants of Galileo, Newton and Descartes needs to pass on to a new generation of innovators. This new generation will acknowledge the truths of reductionistic science but also recognise the limitations and consequences that such a one-sided view of 'natural laws' places on the progress of both man and the planet. The different currents in thought that will influence this new generation are outlined in the next chapter.

2

The Origins of Green Ideas

In attempting to trace the origins of contemporary Green thinking and their link with the practice of medicine, it is important to appreciate how the different approaches to knowledge have influenced both the pace and style of enquiry. From Table 1 we can see that our present concerns form only a small part of the cycle of changes that have occurred on earth. Peter Russell's *The Awakening Earth* draws attention to the specific fields of study that have characterised emergent orders of evolution. (Table 2)

The 'back to nature' aspect of the Green movement draws on a very strong appeal not only in the romantic Rousseau-esque sense but in the writings of nineteenth-century biologists. The founder of modern ecology, Ernest Haekel, was the first to outline some of the guiding principles.[1] Haekel (1834–1919) was a zoologist interested in the microscopic forms of parasitic and amoebic entities. Nevertheless, he was concerned with matters macroscopic and mystical and his two books *The Riddles of the Universe*[2] and *The Wonders of Life*[3] were bestsellers. He coined the term

Table 1 Our present time perspective

Big Bang (formation of universe)		1 January
Formation of Earth		14 September
Origin of life		25 September
Significant oxygen		1 December
First fish		19 December
First mammals		26 December
First humans		31 December
First cave painting	11.59 pm	31 December
Christ	11.59.56 pm	
Renaissance	11.59.59	
Present day	First second of New Year's Day	

Source: C. Sagan *The Dragons of Eden* (1979) (adapted).

Table 2 Emergent orders of evolution, showing fields of study relevant to the different stages. I have termed the state of affairs before the Big Bang the zeroth level, and called it the 'Void'.

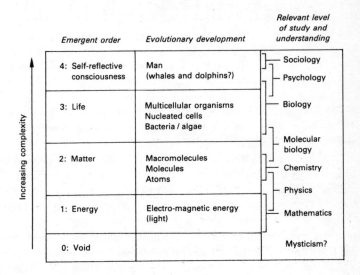

Source: P. Russell *The Awakening Earth* (1982).

'ecology' which he defined as the science of relations between organisms and their environment. His idealism and goal was to search for 'truth' and 'wholeness'.

> While occupying ourselves with the ideal world in art and poetry . . . the real world can be truly known only by experience and pure reason. Truth and poetry are then united in the perfect harmony of monism.[4]

Haekel's ideas and his term ecology were taken up by other biologists including Saint-Hilaire (1854) whose 'fundamental biological notions' included general facts, relationships and organic laws concerning organised beings seen either as whole or via their organs. It is interesting how the words ecology, ethology and economy are often used to describe ordering principles which are seen as necessary for the proper functioning of the universe.

Ethology was at first seen as synonymous with ecology – the battles between the nineteenth-century behaviourists and vitalists later enabled Konrad Lorenz to develop his own understanding of biological ethology, the science of character based on the detailed and precise study of animals. Ecology focused on the physical sphere or energy, climate, plant life and mineral resources, whilst ethology studies the links between animal behaviour, the physical environment and human characteristics. Haekel was a devout and spiritual person, a Monist, who believed 'one spirit in all things, one common fundamental law'. His firm belief in a pantheistic universe was at odds with the monotheistic autocratic religious views he associated with Christianity. He saw Christianity as essentially anti-nature, and was convinced that for Man to live in harmony both with himself and his environment, he had to live by Nature's laws and worship Nature and not an anthropomorphised version of God.

Haekel turned to Buddhism as the one religion that appeared to address the laws on nature – presaging the interest in Eastern philosophy and meditational practices of many participants in today's Green movement. The debate regarding the study of biology which Haekel and his followers commenced has only recently surfaced in medicine. Up until very recently medicine has been content to view man and his diseases from a perspective which is primarily a form of mechanistic materialism and which is in direct contrast to the one now expounded by followers of the Gaia hypothesis and General Systems Theory. And it is from these two separate, though not dissimilar, views of evolutionary theory that Green ideas originate.

The Gaia hypothesis

Formulated by Dr James Lovelock and named after the Greek goddess Gaia, the Earth Mother, it describes the planet as if it were one unitary living system.[5] Lovelock was working on methods of detecting whether living matter existed on planets and developed the hypothesis that if life did exist on a planet it would leave its 'footprints' in the chemical make-up of that planet and that these 'footprints' could be detected over time. In other words, if no life existed, the chemical structure would achieve a state of equilibrium according to physical laws of chemistry, but, if life did exist, it would affect the chemistry of the environment in ways other than could be predicted by physical chemistry alone. Using this principle to study the earth's chemical structure,

Lovelock found that the predicted level of oxygen in the atmosphere would be virtually zero if no life existed on earth. In other words, for life to exist oxygen was required, and if life ceased to exist oxygen would gradually disappear. This symbiotic and homeostatic relationship which had been described in the nineteenth century by Claude Bernard, Lovelock saw as the governing principle in evolutionary progress.

Gaia was the manifestation of the entire range of living matter from viruses through to man, like some giant corporate living entity which in some mysterious way interacts not only with its constituent parts but with the temperature, the atmosphere, the sea and soil to ensure the 'optimum' conditions for the survival of life on the planet.[6] Lovelock went on to identify specific examples of this homeostatic principle including the steadiness of the Earth's surface temperature, the regulation of the amount of salt in the oceans, the stabilisation of the oxygen concentration and the presence of a small quantity of ammonia in the atmosphere. He set up an experiment to test the hypothesis that there are associations of species which co-operate to perform some essential regulatory function, that of keeping the parts of the system related to each other and to the whole. He postulated and identified the presence of carrier compounds for elements essential to all biological systems, iodine and sulphur.

Lovelock gives full credit to earlier scientists for the idea that the earth is a living organism. However it is through his scientific and popular writings that this idea has permeated through much of the Green movement. Lovelock's background is in biology and medicine and it is from the latter discipline that he draws his most evocative metaphors:

Because of this difference in emphasis, a concern for the planet rather than ourselves, I came to realise that there might be the need for a new profession, that of planetary medicine.

At this early stage in our understanding of the Earth as a physiological entity we need General Practitioners, not specialists.

As part of their graduation, physicians must take the Hippocratic Oath. It includes the injunction to do nothing that would harm the patient. A similar oath is needed for the putative planetary doctors if they are to avoid iatrogenic error: an oath to prevent the overzealous from applying a cure that would do more harm than good[7]

Lovelock goes on to give numerous examples of the 'iatrogenic errors' so far applied to the Earth patient. The Gaia hypothesis has been taken up and owned by the Green movement and has, like all cult phenomena, both gained and lost as a result. General Systems Theory, which predates Lovelock's work, has remained more fully within the academic world. Its message, however, is very similar to the Gaia hypothesis, and it has found an increasingly influential place within medicine and biology.

General Systems Theory

Weiss and Von Bertanfly, who are credited with the first exposition of what is now known as General Systems Theory, were biologists who were not afraid to draw on computer and engineering insights in trying to understand their own discipline of biology.[8] Their model of examining the world involved the recognition that nothing could be studied on its own and everything was part of a system.

> A system consists of objects with properties which cohere. The relationships that are brought about by this coherence not only tie the system together, but create conditions from which the properties arise. The importance of the concept of a system is that within an environment a set of objects can be seen to cohere and interact in such a way that their attributes define the nature of the system, and may create properties which the system alone manifests. The coming together to form a system is called systematisation and any tendency of the objects to fall apart is called segregation.

Miller, in his book *Living Systems*, proposed that all living systems are composed of sub-systems.[9] George Engel, the foremost physician to utilise General Systems Theory, advocated a break from the traditional biomedical model with its emphasis on reductionistic and mechanistic thinking that underpins much of the most recent medical advance. Engel labelled his approach to medicine, biopsycho-social and contrasted this with the biomedical model, which he saw as the predominant 'folk-medicine' of Western society. He saw the need to abandon this model as it failed to explain and, more importantly, treat a large proportion of the 'dis-eases' and illnesses that beset Western man.

> The boundaries between health and disease, between well and sick are far from clear and never will be clear for they are diffused by cultural, social and psychological considerations. The traditional biomedical view that biological induces are the ultimate criteria defining disease leads to the present paradox that some people with positive laboratory findings are told they are in need of treatment, when in fact they are feeling quite well, while others feeling sick are assured they are well, that is, they have no disease. A biopsycho-social approach would encompass both circumstances.[10]

Engel drew heavily on Systems Theory to explain and expand on the biopsycho-social approach. He drew on Weiss's statement that nature is ordered both as a hierarchy and a continuum. The components of these models were each given the distinction of a 'system'. Each system or level in the hierarchy possessed distinct characteristics of its own, i.e. a cell operates very differently from a person. Yet each system is a component that can operate as a dynamic whole but at the same time is a component of a higher system, e.g. a cell is part of a tissue and tissues form organs, etc. Thus each system is both a 'whole' and at the same time forms part of a greater whole. It is by exploring the nature of the part and the whole that the 'natural scientist' operates. He is able to dissect and analyse the component parts of any whole – like his reductionistic colleague, but he is aware of the need to see the 'whole' as a 'whole', and also as a part of an even greater whole. It is the dynamic and fluid quality of Systems Theory that allows for a living link to be made between the biological and social sciences. This link has been further strengthened by Prigogine whose concept of dissipative structures won him the Nobel Prize.

> We know we can interact with Nature. That is the heart of the message I give. Matter is not inert. It is alive and active. Life is always changing one way and another through its adaptation to non-equilibrium conditions. With the idea of a doomed permanent world view now gone, we can feel free to make our fate for good or ill. Classical science made us feel that we were helpless witnesses to Newton's clockwork world. Now science allows us to feel at home in nature.

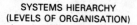

Figure 2 Hierarchy of natural systems

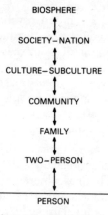

SYSTEMS HIERARCHY
(LEVELS OF ORGANISATION)

BIOSPHERE
↕
SOCIETY – NATION
↕
CULTURE – SUBCULTURE
↕
COMMUNITY
↕
FAMILY
↕
TWO – PERSON
↕

PERSON

(experience and behaviour)

↕
NERVOUS SYSTEM
↕
ORGANS / ORGANS SYSTEMS
↕
TISSUES
↕
CELLS
↕
ORGANELLES
↕
MOLECULES
↕
ATOMS
↕
SUBATOMIC PARTICLES

It is this 'feeling at home in nature' that draws so many of the Green movement together and it is the exposition of these ideas in medicine that George Engel has so elegantly drawn together. Using both models (Figures 2 and 3), he illustrates how the 'systems-orientated physician' can draw on his biochemical knowledge as well as his social and political skills to approach the problems of a middle-aged man with a coronary.[11] In my own paper on the meaning of illness, I further elaborate on Engel's work and describe the 'languages' required by the systems-orientated physician if he/she is to practise 'holistic medicine'.[12] These 'languages' now include: the medical, molecular, material language of classical science; the psychological, psychodynamic and psychosomatic language of Freud, Balint and Grodeck; the

Figure 3 Continuum of natural systems

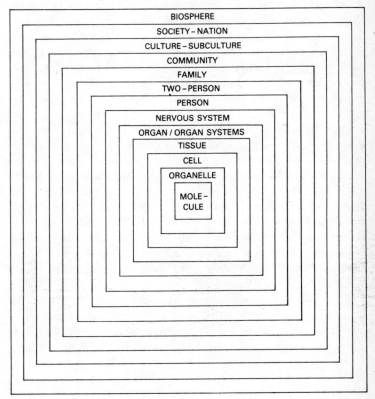

BIOSPHERE
SOCIETY – NATION
CULTURE – SUBCULTURE
COMMUNITY
FAMILY
TWO – PERSON
PERSON
NERVOUS SYSTEM
ORGAN / ORGAN SYSTEMS
TISSUE
CELL
ORGANELLE
MOLE – CULE

cultural, social and political language of Helman, Parsons and
Black; the archetypal, metaphorical and symbolic language of
Jung, Zeidler, Eliade and Hillman; the preventive, educational
and anticipatory language of several official and governmental
reports and, finally, the spiritual, temporal and energetic language found in Eastern medical texts and closely associated with
much of alternative medicine. It is only by adopting a systems
approach where each 'system' and its language can begin to inform
and enrich the others that a truly 'holistic' approach can be
adopted.

Holism and medicine

It is difficult nevertheless not to applaud and indeed stand in awe
of the developments that have occurred in medicine as a result of
the philosophical perspective enunciated so clearly by Descartes
three hundred years ago, and its adopting a predominantly material and molecular language. Like Bacon, who wrote 'We must
put the body on the rack and make it reveal its secrets', the
rationalist doctor became the objective scientific doctor. The wish
to help the patient was overwhelmed by the wish to know. The
role of the doctor as a 'healer' became subordinate to his role as an
objective observer.

Once freed from the Church, medicine made enormous progress. By reducing problems to their smallest part, the discovery
of bacteria, viruses and the molecular nature of disease enabled
doctors to develop treatments which heralded a new age of health
care. With the development of the electron microscope, the
secrets of the chromosome opened up a new vista of genetic
understanding and, more recently, genetic engineering. The
doctor scientist became more and more separated from the 'laws
of nature'. The doctor's task is not to obey or love nature but to
penetrate it, control it and, as we have seen with more recent
medical discoveries, supplant it.

The philosophical debate in medicine, however, was not
altogether one-sided, and the emergence of the concepts of
holism and holistic medicine have attempted to suggest that there
may be another path. Smuts, the South African historian, explorer
and militarist, first coined the term 'holism' in 1926 in his book
Holism and Evolution.[13] He wrote this book in twenty-eight
weeks, as his biographer says, in a mood of 'now or never'.

Essentially his view of holism was not that different to Haekel's use of the word 'ecology' or to the Gaia principle. Smuts defined holism as a 'factor operative towards the making or creating of wholes in the Universe'. He wrote, 'Holism is a factor which underlines the synthetic tendency in the Universe and is the principle which makes for the origin and progress of wholes in the Universe. Wholeness . . . marks the line of evolutionary progress and holism is the inner driving force behind that progress'. Again, we see the link between evolutionary forces and guiding biological principles.

For Smuts, holism did not mean 'the whole is greater than the sum of the parts'. This second definition of holism can be traced to the Gestalt psychologists in the 1920s. Koffka wrote, 'It has been said that the whole is greater than the sum of the parts, because summing is a meaningless procedure whereas whole-part-relationship is meaningful'.[14] Smuts was also fairly careful not to imply the whole is necessarily greater, i.e. better than the part. He wrote, 'It is very important to recognise that the whole is not something additional to the parts. It is the parts in a definitive structural arrangement and with mutual activities which constitute the whole'. Again, one can draw parallels between General Systems Theory and the whole-part relationship emphasised by both Koffka and Smuts. The word holism itself is derived from the Greek word 'holos' meaning whole, complete, and holistic medicine places an emphasis on 'regarding the whole person', body, mind and spirit, and on the whole person within his own system, family, community, culture and environment.

Thus holistic medicine can be seen as applying a General Systems view towards the practice of medicine. Of course 'whole-person' medicine is a concept that all doctors are, or should be, familiar with. But the 'whole' we choose to recognise is too often determined by the prevalent biomedical model, which embraces both reductionism and mind-body dualism. Holistic medicine is indeed about whole-person medicine but its strength and vitality lie in the fact that its definition of what consitutes a 'whole' person is drawn from a number of different disciplines and not solely the biological sciences.[15] It is unfortunate that the term holistic medicine has become almost synonymous with alternative medicine and it is important to distinguish between these two epithets.

Holism espouses an approach and does not dictate any particular therapy. One can be 'holistic' and suggest 'brain surgery' and one can be 'reductive' and treat patients with high doses of vitamin C. The particular therapeutic skill each practitioner employs does not necessarily determine the approach he may take to the problems presented by the patient. The appeal that many 'alternative therapies' have to the Green movement is often based on a misunderstanding of the richness and complexity that underpin the practice of holistic medicine, and has more to do with the search for simple and magical solutions.

What does greening mean?

We have surveyed some of the major conceptual ideas that underpin the 'greening process' and seen how central the shift from *causality* to *connectedness* is. Rather than focus on and search for the causes as to why the universe is as it is, the greening process privileges a perspective which looks for the *connections* that make the universe as it is. The first necessitates a reductionist 'take the clock to bits' approach, the second observes the nature of the clock and how events and people will relate to its function – that of keeping time. In medicine this would imply that rather than focus on the causes of a coronary thrombosis, raised cholesterol, poor oxygen supply, blocked arteries, the focus would be on the circumstances in which the coronary took place, the effect on the patient, and his immediate relatives, the implications regarding work and future relationships etc.

Thus the greening process can be seen as a move towards exploring and developing the connections and relationships we have with

(a) the environment and the world of nature (ecology, environmental concerns, pollution, deforestation, acid rain, lead-free petrol, etc);
(b) other people and other species (feminism, consumerism, animal rights, protection of endangered species);
(c) our 'inner selves' and our 'outer gods' (meditation, consciousness raising, spiritual awareness).

In addition, there is a recognition and an acceptance of the fact that our own existence is determined not only by *our* relationship with those three aspects of our experience, but that there is a reciprocal impact on us, i.e. the environment, other people and our 'gods' influence and affect us in a fundamental way.

Medicine, with its focus on identifying and 'curing' dis-ease, illness and suffering, is intricately involved with many of these issues. As I shall outline in the following chapters, this involvement has now entered a new phase where the problems can no longer be ignored. I shall detail some of these problems first before describing how the greening process has already begun to have an impact on many aspects of medical care.

PART II

The Problems

3

The Magic Bullet Begins to Hurt

Hark the herald angels sing
  Beecham's Pills are just the thing
Peace on earth and mercy mild
  Two for man and one for child[1]

Man has always sought some external substance to take in order to relieve his pain, distress or discomfort. Whether it was a poultice, a liniment, the linctus, some herbal mixture or, literally, the gilded pill. The Egyptians wrapped their medicines in silver or gold leaf, thus ensuring that they were not absorbed in the intestine and passed straight through the person unchanging. The folk healers and white witches of the late middle ages gave way to the apothecaries of the seventeenth century, and the invention of gelatine capsules by French pharmacists in 1834 heralded the beginning of the modern drug industry.[2] Medicines could be delivered in palatable form and be digested and absorbed in the intestine once the gelatine had dissolved.

Gradually the influence of traditional remedies began to lose its hold and the nineteenth-century travelling salesman with his elixir of life beneficial for 'Rheumatiz, Ladies indispositions, Colic, Stones, baldness – also excellent for preserving saddles'[3] gave way to the modern pharmaceutical representative (drug rep.) visiting the doctor and persuading him that his firm's drug for high blood pressure was superior to all the other available drugs. Even though several of the herbal remedies have proved to contain the pharmacological ingredients in many of our modern drugs, fashion and pressure from both the pharmaceutical and medical professions has ensured that the prescribing of drugs has become the preferred method of treatment. Reading through some of the folk remedies for sore throats one can understand why it has become more acceptable to take a pill: 'For sore throat, swallow a teaspoon of sugar saturated with turpentine or Kerosene or blow dry sulphur through a paper funnel.'[4]

With the formation of the British Medical Association in the nineteenth century, some attempt was made to regulate and license proprietary preparations and patent medicines. The drug explosion and the belief in the magic bullet as a solution to man's ills did not really commence until the beginning of the twentieth century. The discovery of quinine, sulphonamides, vitamins and finally antibiotics heralded an era where it appeared as if our scientists and pharmacists would indeed find 'a pill for every ill'. With the advent of the National Health Service (NHS) in 1949 and the availability of free prescriptions, the use of folk remedies and non-pharmaceutical methods decreased. Parallel with this decrease, an escalating increase in drug-prescribing and drug-taking developed.

At present, nearly 12 per cent of all NHS expenditure is attributable to drugs. Currently this figure is about £2,000,000 a year; more than the cost of all general practitioners and community services. Even when taking inflation into account, the cost of GP prescribing is five times more than it was in 1949 when the NHS was first established. This shift in behaviour has been accompanied, and, some would say, actively encouraged by the drug industry. This branch of our national life has become one of the most successful industries in the United Kingdom, employing over 70,000 people a year and contributing around £700 million to Britain's balance of trade figures through its exports.[5]

As general practitioners issue over 75 per cent of all prescribed drugs used, the drug companies aim their promotional material at the GP through advertising, direct mail, sponsorship and direct influence via the drug rep. This represents an expenditure of about £7,000 a year on every GP in this country and, as each GP prescribes about £70,000 worth of drugs, it is a reasonable investment. Once qualified, most doctors attempt to keep up-to-date through reading medical journals or attending meetings, but over 40 per cent of the information which influences their decision as to what to prescribe is received by them directly from drug companies.[6] Drug reps visit GPs in their offices, often offering them lunch or some 'inducement', a new blood pressure machine or a computer for example, and will discuss with them the benefits of prescribing their particular drug. Doctors are given free samples and on some occasions will be offered a financial inducement for every patient recruited to take part in a 'research trial'. Some of these gross abuses have been dropped by the drug industry's own code of practice, but they remain a powerful and subtle way of influencing doctors' prescribing habits. It would be fair to say that similar techniques are used in the 'alternative field'. Any journal or magazine on health-care carries with it glossy ads on this or that food, nutrient, mineral supplement, 'natural' health and/or bionic lamp, all promising relief for a whole host of symptoms.

We live in a consumer society and drugs as well as 'natural medicine' are very big business, which attracts all the talents and skills of marketing. The drug industry has been particularly successful in securing the market place and almost imprisoning the suppliers to the public (doctors), so that on occasion it may appear that doctors are no more than paid agents of the drug industry. Many doctors would rightfully resent this implication, but until medical education is broadened, doctors' ability to choose the appropriate treatment will be severely limited.

Clearly the consumer has had a willing and at times encouraging part to play in this increase. At any one time, 60 per cent of the population will be taking a drug of some kind and only half will have had this drug prescribed by their doctors.[7] These over-the-counter drugs (o.t.c.) are obtained for many of the minor and self-limiting conditions that human beings are prone to. Their sales were not affected by the onset of the NHS and relatively free prescriptions, and most households stock at least one proprietary medicine.

The national characteristics of self-medication reveal major differences both in quantity of drugs consumed as well as type.

Table 3 Households with various medicines

Medicine	Households %
Analgesics	85
Ointments etc.	54
Indigestion mix.	35
Cough medicine	35
Laxatives	43
Iron, Vitamins	29

Source: K. Dunnell & A. Cartwright *Medicine Takers, Prescribers and Hoarders* (1972).

Vitamins and minerals are consumed by 59 per cent of children and 29 per cent of adults in Helsinki compared with 8 per cent in Buenos Aires and 2 per cent in Yugoslavia. At any one time 16 per cent of people in Liverpool are taking laxatives whilst only 2 per cent of Yugoslavs consume these drugs.[8] The French like their suppositories and liver pills, the English like their cough medicines and linctuses.

It is not only in over-the-counter sales that we can see these national trends. Treating *low* blood pressure, a condition not described in medical text-books other than as a result of a medical emergency, varies from country to country. (Table 4.) Fashion in prescribing amongst doctors is as common a feature as in the motor-car industry. In 1960 over 25 per cent of prescriptions for osteo-arthritis were for Butazolidin, a drug not approved in the United States and subsequently banned in the UK.

Over 6,500 preparations are available for prescribing in the UK compared with 1,900 in Norway, even though the World Health Organisation has only 250 essential drugs on its list.[9] The development of new chemical entities (NCE) within drug companies appears to be more related to commercial pressures than to pharmaceutical advances. Of the 204 NCEs introduced between 1971 and 1980 in the UK, it was claimed that the majority were for 'common or largely chronic conditions'.[10] In the USA, the Food & Drugs Administration rates each new drug A (important), B (modest therapeutic value), C (little or no gain). Out of every 20 new drugs that appear on the market each year one was rated A, three were B and 16 were C.[11] The arguments that the drug companies rehearse include the fact that the amount of investment required to discover a really important drug is huge and without the commercial sales or 'loss leaders' they could not

Table 4 Prescriptions written for hypotension (i.e. to raise blood pressure) in 1974, per 1 million population

Country	No. of prescriptions	Country	No. of prescriptions
UK	200	Spain	39,000
Holland	4,100	Italy	102,200
Belgium	9,300	Japan	104,400
France	20,900	Germany	154,000

Source: Source of Information for Prescribing Doctors in Britain, O.H.E. (1977).

survive. The problem would not be so acute if their products were generally harmless.

Drugs and their dangers

The tragedy of modern medical education is that most doctors and increasingly most patients believe that treatment requires the prescription of one or other drug. The consequences of this collusion would be less serious were it not for the danger of modern drugs. Drugs are powerful chemicals and their dangers arise from a number of factors other than their side-effects. Incautious and grossly negligent prescribing on the part of doctors still occurs more frequently than it should. Over 50,000 prescriptions in a teaching hospital in the US were analysed to reveal over-medication (too much or too frequent use) in one in eight prescriptions. A number of the drugs prescribed together were known to have harmful interaction.[12] Doctors' illegible handwriting has landed them in court and their patients in hospital. The frequency and use of repeat prescriptions written by receptionist staff have added to the number of mistakes or overdosage. The recent introduction of computers within general practice has been seen as a way of minimising these human errors, but the wrong medicine for the wrong person continues to be prescribed.

Once patients are prescribed drugs, they may fail to have them dispensed (10–15 per cent) or they may fail to comply with the instructions and, more commonly, they stop the course of treatment sooner than the doctor suggested. It is estimated that at least two out of five never take their prescribed drugs,[13] and the hoarding of drugs suggests this may even be higher. In 1976, 200,000 tablets were returned during a 'drug amnesty' in the small area of Dudley, Hereford and Worcester; in 1979 this figure rose to 300,000, and in 1982 it was 740,000.[14] More serious than the non-compliance is the faulty compliance where patients, especially the elderly, fail to understand the instructions and either take too many or combine the wrong drugs from previous prescriptions. Every year over 200,000 adults and children are admitted to hospital because of an overdose of some kind, accidental or otherwise. Four thousand people a year die from drug overdose and at any one time it is estimated that one in six hospital admissions are there because of some side-effect of their medication.[15]

Side-effects are part and parcel of any drug effect. The usual way for the medical profession to assess the danger of a drug is to calculate its risk/benefit ratio. Does the risk of taking the drug outweigh the benefit derived from it? Drugs are extensively tested before being released on the market and through a system of reporting (Yellow Card), doctors inform the Committee on Safety of Medicines of possible dangerous side-effects. Nevertheless, tragedies continue to occur, as evidenced by the consequences following the prescribing of thalidomide, Opren, chloramphenicol, Butazolidin.

It is not solely the misuse of drugs and their potential side-effects that give rise for concern. One of the most plangent criticisms against the medical profession was outlined by Ivan Illich. In his book *Medical Nemesis* (later retitled *Limits to Medicine*), he castigated the profession for encouraging the 'medicalisation' of many of life's natural processes (pregnancy, birth, marriage, death, sexual intercourse etc).[16] He felt that the 'promise' to end all pain and eliminate disease was a tragic dehumanising confidence-trick. He suggested that most traditional healing methods were a way of consoling, caring and comforting people as the natural process of healing occurs. By its highly interventionist approach, medicine was robbing people of their ability to experience and make tolerable pain, sickness, impairment and death. Illich felt that the word 'suffering' had taken on a sado-masochistic flavour which for many traditional cultures not touched by Western medicine was not present. 'Patience, tolerance, courage, resignation, self-control, perseverance and meekness: each expresses a different colouring of the responses with which pain sensations were accepted, transformed into the experience of suffering and endured.' The loss of these responses has led to a diminution of human endeavour so that we arrive at a situation where we do expect a 'pill for every ill'. Illich labelled this transformation of cultural responses 'a cultural iatrogenesis'. His arguments, because they appeared so general and one-sided, have not been taken very seriously and his book has largely been ignored by the medical profession.

Illich's descriptions may well be accurate but he failed to see that this cultural iatrogenesis arises out of a collusion between doctor and patients. We, as patients, make demands on our doctors to 'take the pain away'. 'Can't you cure me doctor?' The initial successes of modern pharmacology have made it seem as if

Figure 4 Average NHS prescriptions each person per annum

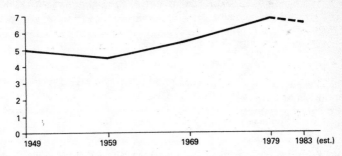

Source: J. Fry, D. Brock, I. McColl *et al.*, *NHS Data Book* (1984).

this state of affairs might really come about. Doctors were all too happy to play their part and appear as man's saviour. The result of this collusion is the enormous increase in prescribing that now consumes over 12 per cent of the total health budget. Nevertheless it is possible to discern large cultural and regional variations in prescribing patterns. The UK national pattern of prescribing has increased from 4.9 prescriptions per person per year to 6.5 prescriptions per year. Based on international comparisons British patients receive significantly fewer prescriptions from their doctors per capita per year (6.5) than patients in Japan (35), France

Figure 5

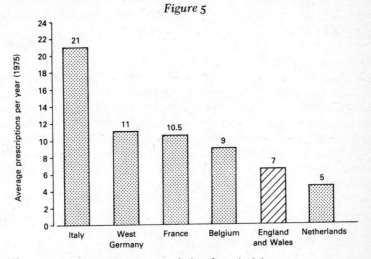

Source: C. Medawar, *The Wrong Kind of Medicine* (1984).

Table 5 Patients' expectations of doctor's actions

Action expected	Percentage of patients
Prescription only	51.4
Prescription and sickness certificate	6.9
Prescription and other	2.8
Sickness certificate only	9.7
Other (results, opinion, minor surgery)	12.5
Not sure what to expect	16.7

Source: G. C. Stimson and B. Webb, *Going to see the Doctor* (1975).

(10) and Spain (9.6). Similarly British doctors are more conservative than their colleagues in other EC and developed countries when it comes to prescribing new products. In the UK in 1987, only 9.3 per cent of total pharmaceutical prescriptions by value were for new products, compared to France (13.3%), Holland (15.7%), Germany (16.6%) Italy (29.3%), Japan (25.8%) and the USA (22.1%). In comparison with other European countries we give ourselves far fewer prescriptions per person in one year. Within the UK even wider variations can be found. Figures are at times hard to come by but on average about 80 per cent of all consultations in General Practice will end with a prescription. The interesting fact to note is that when patients are asked before the consultation, 60 per cent will be expecting a prescription.[17] (Table 5.) Some GPs, those who are members of the Royal College of General Practitioners, will prescribe on average 54 per cent of the time, and several studies have identified even lower prescribing rates.[18] The reasons for these regional variations may vary, e.g. because of the age of the population, thus elderly patients are issued with, on average, 15 prescriptions per year. A study undertaken in 1985 demonstrated a linear relationship between high rates of unemployment and high rates of prescribing.[19] Department of Health statistics show that the highest rate of prescribing was in the North West of England (unemployment 13.4%) and the lowest rate of prescribing was in the North West Thames area (unemployment 7.5%).

It is thus clear that the act of prescribing is a much more complex medical activity than simply giving a patient a pharmacologically active drug which is hoped will effect the course of the disease. Some of the possible non-pharmacological functions of prescribing are listed in Table 6. The Greenfield Report[20] on effective prescribing made major recommendations regarding the training of doctors and felt that, in general, in the instructions given to medical students and trainee general practitioners a balance was lacking between pharmacology (the study of drugs) and therapeutics (the treatment of disease). The writing of a prescription is one of the stages in most consultations, and forms a vehicle for communication with the patient. It is a legal document and the medical profession guards its monopoly on prescribing with great care.

Moves to allow nurses to prescribe a range of simple drugs have always been resisted, and unlike other European countries, the sale of most drugs direct to the patient is strictly limited.

The most quoted of the reasons for prescribing non-drugs is the placebo effect. A much misused term and poorly understood mechanism, the placebo effect has kept health-care practitioners of all kinds in business for centuries. It is usually defined in the medical literature as a pharmacologically inert substance – only a placebo – yet its power to cure and heal has consistently been found to be present in 30–40 per cent of all diseases, no matter what their severity, including angina and schizophrenia.[21] Rather than build on this naturally given therapeutic process, it is often

Table 6 Some possible hidden functions of the prescription

- Visible sign of the doctor's power to heal
- Symbol of the power of modern technology
- Sign that the patient is 'really ill'
- Concrete expression that doctor has fulfilled his or her contract
- Reasonable excuse for human contact with doctor
- Satisfactorily terminates the visit
- Fits the concept that modern humans can control their own destiny
- Expression of doctor's control
- Indication of doctor's concern
- Medium of communication between doctor and patient
- Forestalls lengthy discussions
- Source of satisfaction to the doctor
- Identifies the clinical situation as legitimately medical
- Legitimises sick role status
- Symbol of patient control
- Means of patient goal attainment

Source: Based on M. Smith in R. E. A. Mapes *Prescribing Practice and Drug Usage* (1980).

dismissed both by doctors and patients. It is the *belief* of those both receiving and giving the intervention (placebo need not always be a drug) that determines its efficacy, and the reason for introducing double-blind trials in research studies is to control for this effect. In a well-known study, it was shown that there is a consistent pattern of about 70–90 per cent effectiveness reported initially by enthusiasts of a particular form of therapy, be it a drug, a psychological intervention or alternative therapy. When 'non-enthusiasts' or sceptics use the similar therapy, the effectiveness is reduced to 30–40 per cent.[21] It is not only the patient's faith in the therapy that is important; it is the doctor's as well. In another study on asthma, the doctor conducting the study found that patients improved on the active drug but not on the placebo. Unknown to the doctor the active drug had been substituted with another placebo. The positive effect on the patient was the result of the doctor's belief that he was prescribing a drug and not just a placebo.[22] For effective treatment to take place, both doctor and patient need to share a belief that the treatment prescribed will work. The placebo effect can be influenced by a number of factors including the colour of the pill. Anxiety symptoms are best treated with green pills, depressive symptoms with yellow pills and pain symptoms with red pills.[23] Patients with headaches responded much better to 'brand names' advertised on television than to a similar drug which was not so well-known. The authority of the prescriber (white coat, stethoscope), increases the placebo effect, as does the personality of the receiver. Attributes of the 'placebo personality' include 'over-anxiety, emotional dependence and immaturity'.[24]

Methods of regulating and monitoring the development of new medicines together with attempts to influence the way doctors prescribe have only recently been introduced. Following the thalidomide disaster, the Medicines Act was passed and two groups, the Committee on Safety of Medicines (all new products) and the Committee for the Review of Medicines (CRM) were set up. These committees recommended to the licensing authority (DHSS) whether or not a licence for a new or existing drug should be granted. Drug companies could appeal against any ruling to the Medicines Commission. In addition, the Dunlop Committee on Safety of Medicines recommended the use of the Yellow Card system. Yellow cards, however, are filled in infrequently, approximately 12,000 a year – one card per GP every two years, which does not suggest that this early warning system operates effectively. Even the close monitoring of the official committees has not prevented several new drugs having to be withdrawn within a few years of their release, as a result of mounting evidence of their dangers. Obtaining compensation from drug companies involves many years of hard work and tedious legal hearings, which can take ages to process. Moreover, in Britain, unlike America, there have been no recorded cases of patients successfully suing drug companies. AMVA (Action for the Victims of Medical Accidents), the Opren Action Group and APVDC (Association of Parents of Vaccine Damaged Children) have around 1,500 individual cases awaiting the results of litigation against drug companies. To this figure must now be added a growing group of patients claiming damages from the lengthy prescribing of psychotropic drugs (Valium, Mogadon, etc).

Attempts by the medical profession to influence the prescribing of drugs involve sending GPs regular information. These publications include *The British National Formulary*, *Prescribers Journal* and the *Drug & Therapeutics Bulletin*. The DoH employs Independent Medical Advisers to visit GPs whose prescribing policies appear to be out of the ordinary. These visits usually occur when a GP's drug bill exceeds 20 per cent of the national average.

Accurate figures for each doctor's prescribing costs have been available for a number of years and with the recent introduction of the Prescribing Analyses and Cost (PACT) system, it is now possible to determine exactly which group of drugs, e.g. sleeping tablets, antibiotics, are being over-prescribed. Harris, in his study of prescribing habits, found that simply by providing GPs with this detailed knowledge, their prescribing habits could be influenced.[25] This was especially true as to whether they used generic names (diazepam) or the brand name (Valium) on their prescription. The Greenfield Committee (1982) recommended that generic prescribing should become the norm and that new products should not be given a brand name. It has been estimated that the drug bill would be reduced by 10 per cent. Drug companies understandably have fought a major campaign against the introduction of generic prescribing, identifying some legitimate areas of concern, which include lack of adequate controls, poor quality testing, decreased patient compliance and confidence. Nevertheless, there has been a steady reduction in the percentage of drugs prescribed using their brand names. A further attempt to regulate and reduce the number of drugs available on prescription was the introduction of the selected lists. In 1985, a group of professional medical advisers drew up a selected list of drugs for seven therapeutic groups. These included tranquillisers, hypnotics, minor analgesics, cough suppressants, antacids, laxatives and vitamins. Doctors are only allowed to prescribe from this limited list on the NHS prescription. They are free to prescribe what they choose if the drug is not included on this list, e.g. antibiotics. Following the introduction of this list, many doctors felt it would limit their clinical freedom. This does not seem to have occurred and an increasing number of hospital pharmacies and group practices are producing their own list of 'approved' drugs.

Although both the medical profession and the pharmaceutical industry are often seen as the causes for the increasing use of drugs, it would be inaccurate to blame them or to look for sinister motives. We need look no further than ourselves. If we insist on renewing our cars every two to three years, buying the latest electronic toy and responding to the dictates of fashion, we then also demand new drugs, the miracle cure – and the magic bullet. In this most consumer of ages we prefer to buy tablets for our high blood pressure, antacids for our ulcers and antibiotics for our colds. The fact that our blood pressure could possibly be controlled by a relaxation exercise practised daily, or our ulcer symptoms by a change of diet, and that colds are not responsive to antibiotics does not impress us, for it is much easier to take a pill than change our life-style or accept the limitations of everyday life. It is far easier to place the causes of much of our illnesses on external factors than to accept some responsibility ourselves for their occurrence.

The 'greening process', with its emphasis on 'natural' life-styles and a bias against the taking of drugs, may be thought to have influenced prescribing patterns. As yet, there is no hard evidence of any major shift amongst either doctors or patients. The shift, if there has been one, is towards a greater ingestion of supplemental vitamins, minerals and tablets thought not to be 'drugs', e.g. Evening Primrose Oil, Germanium. The reliance on the 'magic bullet' approach appears to be as high as ever: there is, though, a search for a magic bullet that doesn't hurt quite so much as the ones produced by pharmaceutical companies.

4

The Tyranny of Excellence

Over the last hundred or so years medicine has made progress as a result of the willingness to espouse a scientific approach to the understanding and treatment of illness. The Cartesian model of the human body has influenced the development of the objective analytic doctor. Indeed for a doctor to claim he was unscientific would ensure that his opinions would be dismissed. Science, as perceived by medicine, involved objective measurement, a preference for unitary causes of diseases – one kind of bacteria causes one infection which is cured by one antibiotic – and a fascination with instrumentation and technology that is the mainstay of most modern Western hospitals. This approach – the biomedical model – has led to the increasing specialisation and compartmentalisation of the patient, with the concomitant distancing and devaluing of the human element in the transaction between doctor and patient. Doctors, it seems, would be much happier to study diseases than actually to treat patients. And yet, until fairly recently, the premise on which medicine lays claim to being scientific appears to have gone unchallenged. The definition of what constitutes science and the scientific method is hotly debated even amongst the 'pure' scientists themselves. Sir Peter Medawar wrote:

> Ask a scientist what he conceives the scientific method to be and he will adopt an expression that is at once solemn and shifty-eyed, solemn because he feels he ought to declare an opinion, shifty-eyed because he is wondering how to conceal the fact that he has no opinion to declare. If taunted he would probably mumble something about 'induction' and 'establishing the laws of nature', but if anyone working in a laboratory professed to be trying to establish the laws of nature by induction we should begin to think he was overdue for leave.[1]

The 'scientific method' as it has evolved includes *causality* – 'how to connect elements known to be associated with one another in the correct way' – and that correct way involves looking for a logical sequence of cause and effect.

'The notion of causality pervades the whole of science and no one science has any special claim to adjudicate upon its usage.' By this is meant that a logical sequence exists between the moment a blow is imparted to a billiard ball and its final resting place. With the proper measuring instruments and accurate information on the force imparted, the size and shape of the ball, the surface of the billiard table, the angle at which the force is delivered etc, it is possible to predict where that final resting place will be. Most of Western science relies on the discovery of 'natural laws' which allow for accurate and repeatable predictions as to why 'things' happen and how causality can be accurately determined. The possibility that other 'theories of causality' exist in the philosophy of scientific thought, and that these theories may also be useful in explaining and predicting human behaviour is not a possibility that many doctors entertain. Jung's idea of the 'acausal connecting principle' which he later termed synchronistic principle is also found in much Chinese thinking and medical practice. This is best stated by Joseph Needham and labelled the nature of 'co-relative and co-ordinate relationships'.

> Things behave in particular ways, not necessarily because of prior actions or impulsions of other things but because their position in the ever moving cyclical universe was such that they were endowed with intrinsic natures which made their behaviour inevitable for them.
>
> The idea of correspondence has greater significance and replaces the idea of causality for things are *connected* and not caused.[2]

Again we observe how connectedness is seen to be of more significance than causation. This theme of connectedness runs through much of 'green' philosophic thought and was outlined earlier in the descriptions of Gaia, Systems Theory and Holism. It is interesting to note that the insights derived from sub-atomic physics and latterly, the theory of chaos, have led the most eminent of Western scientists to declare almost heretical statements regarding the nature of the universe.

Niels Bohr

The great extension of our experience in recent years has brought to light the insufficiency of our simple mechanical conceptions and as a consequence has shaken the foundation on which the customary interpretation of observations was based.

Werner Heisenberg

Nothing is more important about the quantum principle than this, that it destroys the concept of the world 'sitting out there'. To describe what has happened one has to cross out the old word observer and put in its place the new word participator! In some strange sense the universe is a participatory universe.

Illya Prigogine

We know we can interact with nature. That is the heart of the message I give. Matter is not inert. It is alive and active. Life is always changing one way or another through its adaptation to non-equilibrium conditions. With the idea of a doomed determinist world view now gone, we can feel free to make our fate for good or ill. Classical science made us feel that we were helpless witnesses to Newton's clockwork world. Now a science allows us to feel at home in nature.

David Bohm

Ultimately the entire universe (with all its 'particles' including those constituting human beings, their laboratories, observing instruments etc) has to be understood as a single undivided whole, in which analysis into separately and independently existing paths has no fundamental status.

It is, however, important to avoid the pitfall of 'quantum silliness' and remember that mechanistic explanations of cause and effect, although no longer foolproof, still allow us to understand the majority of the phenomena we encounter in everyday life. However, where the idea of 'connectedness' as opposed to causality can lead to greater insights and truths as opposed to facts is in medical practice itself.

For the importance of causality to medicine cannot be overstated, for on this understanding so much of diagnosis, treatment and research is based. The concepts of 'connectedness' and 'patterning' appear at odds with a linear causal model. This difference can best be observed in the diagnostic processes employed by doctors.

The diagnostic process can be defined 'as the acquisition of information about the person's condition which provides a basis for future management and which actually includes a predictive element'. As described by Elstein it involves four sequential stages, 'the collection of data' (history, physical examination, investigation)[3], 'data interpretation', 'hypothesis generation', and 'hypothesis evaluation'. The process is not dissimilar to the inductive reasoning as outlined by Bacon – according to 'inductivism' the doctor should begin 'from scratch' to assemble all the data first, before deciding on the diagnosis. This is still the preferred and taught method at medical school. It is seen to be the 'most scientific' and the dictum 'Diagnosis first, treatment second' ensures that the need for diagnostic accuracy may be pursued, with painful and invasive investigations, long after there is any clear benefit to the patient in terms of treatment. It is clear that even though the process of inductive reasoning still holds sway in the teaching of medical students, many doctors, including 'expert clinicians', have abandoned this model and would appear to operate much closer to the 'hypothetico-deductive model' that became established by the late nineteenth century. Thus Crombie found that, in over 300 consecutive consultations, a specific medical diagnosis 'was arrived at in only 150 and that "treatment" was commenced even though the problem presented would not "fit" any of the classical medical diagnoses'.[4] Elstein in his own survey on the diagnostic process found that 'expert clinicians' formulated a tentative hypothesis within the first few seconds of a consultation, used a form of 'pattern-recognition' in obtaining information and relied on a series of highly discriminate questions to test their original hypothesis. A general practitioner faced on a home visit with a young girl with right-sided abdominal pain has to make the decision to leave her at home or to admit her to hospital. Whether she has appendicitis or not is only part of his concern: he will take other factors into account – the level of anxiety (both his and the parents'), the home circumstances, what time of day or night it is, whether he is on call over the whole weekend, what his own level of confidence is, etc – before deciding whether or not to admit the girl to hospital. The surgeon seeing the young girl in casualty has to decide: 'Do I operate or not?', and he will have to take into account another set of data, 'Has she eaten?', 'Is the anaesthetist busy?', is he confident enough of the diagnosis of appendicitis? The pathologist who is asked to examine the specimen will examine the slides and arrive at a decision on whether the girl had appendicitis or not, relying on a completely different set of 'data'. All three doctors have to decide whether or not the girl has appendicitis, but each arrives at this decision using different sets of information. All information-gathering is value-laden and the notion of the objective scientific doctor using pure induction to arrive at his diagnosis has done much to undermine the medical students' training. The need to be seen to be scientific would not be so problematic if medicine's view of what constitutes science was not so patently out of date, and ironically, so un-scientific. Karl Popper explains:

> The belief that we can start with pure observations alone, without anything in the nature of a theory is absurd as may be illustrated by the story of the man who dedicated his life to natural science, wrote down everything he could observe, and bequeathed his priceless collection of observations to the Royal Society to be used as inductive evidence. This story should show us that though beetles may be profitably collected, observations may not.[5]

The need to be seen as 'scientific' is so great amongst doctors that it is difficult to prise them away from an outmoded view of science, and confusion abounds between science as a 'method of enquiry' and science as a 'body of knowledge'. The epithet 'scientific' is used to denote that it is an acceptable subject for doctors to study. This narrow and inaccurate conception of science within medicine has led to a promulgation of measurement and measuring instrumentation, so that more 'knowledge = science' can be obtained – the more measurements there are the better. The more detailed and complex the measuring instruments required to obtain these measurements the better, so that doctors become the possessors of 'esoteric knowledge', which they alone can own, and which ensures that the patient is kept at a distance both as the object of the measurements and because of his inability to make any sense of them. The development of 'high-tech' medicine which follows this fascination for precision and excellence has led to the development of medical care that still remains unchallenged. Comparative large-scale random surveys comparing the benefits to patients with coronaries nursed in intensive-care units and at home have shown no difference in morbidity or mortality. Yet intensive-care units require three times more equipment and five times more nursing staff than normal care. Even at the other end of the scale of technology, a World Health Organisation survey on the impact of a foetal monitor in the obstetric services of a Third World country showed that the consequences were far from beneficial and indeed were positively harmful. Both the public and governments alike collude with the medical profession in a continuing macabre fascination with high-tech medicine. As has been suggested by Illich, the collusion can be understood as a deep-seated need for the engineering of miracles. 'Intensive care is but the culmination of a public worship organised around a medical priesthood struggling against death.'[6]

Clinical trials

In the BMA report on *Alternative Therapy*, the major criticism levelled against such therapies was that they were 'unscientific'. The definition of the scientific method was the one already referred to earlier in this chapter – 'namely the systematic observation of natural phenomena for the purposes of discovering laws governing those phenomena'.[7] The report defines the scientific approach of validation to include the 'normally approved method of the clinical trial'. It is the 'clinical trial' as a method of assessing the validified treatments that has governed the rules of research in medicine and that has, by and large, determined the progress of Western medicine in the last twenty years. Improvements and advances in clinical medicine have arisen partly from 'trial and error', partly from 'intuitive hunches' and partly from systematic observation and study. Many new treatments which are heralded as 'breakthrough' by their proposers are found to be either useless, dangerous or both. Clinical medicine has a long history of these treatments which become fashionable, sometimes for decades, before being discarded. Tonsillectomies were commonly undertaken for three decades before it became clear that they were of limited use in the management of tonsillitis. The degree to which diagnosis is biased towards illness and the performance of unnecessary surgery was revealed in a study undertaken in 1934, although it took another thirty years before the wide-scale use of this operation decreased. The study revealed that of 1,000 eleven-year-old children in New York, 61 per cent had had their tonsils removed. The remaining 39 per cent were examined by a new panel of doctors and 45 per cent of these were recommended to have a tonsillectomy. The rejected group were re-examined by another panel of doctors and a further 46 per cent were recommended to have surgery.[8]

More recently, radical mastectomies for the treatment of breast cancer were found to be no better than simple mastectomies and radiotherapy but not before thousands of women had been subjected to grotesquely mutilating operations. Other discarded treatments have included colectomy for 'intestinal stasis', a common diagnosis in the Twenties. More recently, the wide-scale use of Caesarean section, hysterectomies and coronary by-pass operations have all been questioned. The rationale for the establishment of a strict 'clinical trial' is to avoid such errors and to allow for a more rational approach to the assessment of claims made for one form of treatment as opposed to another. 'So before embarking indiscriminately on any novel conventional treatment, we must always ask "How do we know that this works?"'[9]

One does not have to be a doctor or a scientist to share the commonsense sentiments in this remark, and the development of the clinical trial is the attempt by the medical profession to address this question. Examples of early 'trials' were the observations by Semmelweiss in 1857 that soaking the hands in disinfectant solution before examining patients in the delivery room reduced the death rate from 18 per cent to 1–2 per cent. In 1930 Louis was able to demonstrate, using large numbers of patients, that blood-letting with leeches was useless as a form of treatment. The more modern approach to clinical trials began when Sir Bradford Hill first tried streptomycin for the treatment of tuberculosis in 1946, but it was not until the late Sixties and Seventies that the randomised controlled trial became the 'normally approved method' for the assessment of new treatments. The methodology adopted for organising such trials has been refined over the last ten years and the current practice includes some if not all of the following features. The patients taking part in such a trial are *randomised*, i.e. they are either allocated to the new treatment group or the control group in a random fashion. There is a *control* group which receives no new treatment and possibly sham or placebo treatment. The patients are not told which group they have been allocated to (*single blind*) and ideally the doctors undertaking the treatment are also unaware as to whether the patient is in the treatment group or the placebo group (*double blind*). There is a *follow-up* period after the trial to evaluate both long-term results and possible side-effects to the new treatment. So that the ideal trial is one which is randomised, controlled, double-blind with long-term follow-up. It is clearly not possible to ensure all these aspects in every trial but the current yardstick of 'excellence' and scientific precision is thought to require all the features thus described. The development of the clinical trial as has been noted arose out of laudable aims, but the consequence of the methodology now adopted and sought for by most of the major research grant-giving bodies has had unforeseen results in terms of clinical progress, patient participation, ethical implications and conceptual understanding as to the nature of health and illness.

Critics have suggested that random selection of trial subjects cannot be achieved – human beings, unlike engines on a test bed, are infinitely variable and unique. The process of randomisation does not produce the homogeneity sought for and does not allow for the generalisation from one group to another. The process, to be precise, requires a limitation of the variables measured both before and after the trial, which belies and denies the infinitely variable nature of human responses. The pursuit of certainty, like the pursuit of excellence and precision, blinds the doctor to a method of working which becomes blind to the paradox that 'all exact science is dominated by the idea of approximation'.

A further consequence of the pursuit of the precise is that all too quickly the patient can get in the way, and the researchers and clinicians are in danger of losing touch with the patients' needs. 'The random and blind assignment of persons to treatment and control groups which is the fundamental basis of this inquiry method . . . fails to treat people holistically. More than this a medical practice which bases its knowledge on this kind of inquiry will inevitably create a culture of alienation. Such a culture will alienate the patient from what is going on in her body and from decisions about treatment.'[10] The authors of this view go on to suggest that rather than try to control for the subjectivity of both patient and researcher (an impossible task in their view), the very powerful nature of this subjectivity should be acknowledged, catered for and included *in* the research design and evaluated as part of the treatment effect. They conclude that the orthodox research designs represent a fragmented empiricism which is incapable of taking persons as wholes.

The greening process is not only about a shift in the things we do – it requires a shift in the way we think. The conceptual understanding of the relationship between part and whole (man and his environment, a diseased organ and the person) forms the basis of the Gaia hypothesis, General Systems theory and holistic medicine. These ways of thinking allow for an approach to research that is fundamentally different from that which is practised by the majority of medical scientists.

The nature of scientific inquiry and its limitations has been a point of debate and exploration amongst 'pure' scientists and 'social' scientists for several decades. The medical profession, which is so well-placed between both extremes, has, for the most part, not entered the debate, and has attempted to resolve the conflict by identifying with the 'pure' form of analytic science, which strives to reject the indeterminate, relies on Aristotelian logic and considers the nature of scientific knowledge to be impersonal, value free, precise and reliable. The analytic scientist's approach to 'knowledge' can be contrasted to that held by the Particular Humanist:

> The Particular Humanist naturally treats every human being as though he or she were unique, not to be compared with anyone or anything else. Thus the Particular Humanist is not interested in formulating general theories of human behaviour at all – not so much because this is impossible (although the Particular Humanist argues it is impossible) but because it is not desirable. To study people in general, even from a humanistic perspective, is for the Particular Humanist inevitably to lose sight of the unique humanity of an individual – to fail to capture precisely *this* person. The Particular Humanists take to heart Kant's dictum to treat everyone as a unique means rather than an abstract theoretical end.[11]

The Particular Humanist's view of scientific knowledge is that it is personal, value-constituted, partisan, non-rational and political. This point of view, so opposite in view to the Analytic Scientist's, does not occupy a privileged position within the practice of medicine, but can be found in both novels and poems. Medical men who have written and revealed truths about the practice of medicine not found in any scientific journal include Chekov, Asher, Sacks and Abse. These truths and insights are as relevant and often far more long-lasting than those identified through a double-blind controlled trial.

That medical students receive so little encouragement, and are, indeed, often discouraged from developing this approach to the study of people, has impoverished medicine as a discipline, and has, as a consequence, contributed to the ethical dilemmas that beset so many of the more recent developments in medical care. Doctors have been so unusued to considering the 'uniqueness of each individual patient' that the longest hearing in the history of the GMC Disciplinary Committee arose as a result of three senior and eminent surgeons and physicians being charged with unprofessional conduct for taking part in the purchase of kidneys from Turkish peasants for use in a private hospital transplant programme. It is an inevitable consequence of the hold that the 'analytic scientific' point-of-view has on medicine that the ethics regarding research trials in in-vitro fertilisation, embryo research, transplant surgery, genetic engineering, and other new developments are having to be debated and discussed mostly by people outside the profession. The ethical and moral dilemmas facing the analytic scientific doctor start with the randomised controlled trial – the 'normally approved method' for undertaking medical research. Glaring examples of the problems that arise if the need to know is determined by this chosen method occurred in the use of placebo tablets in testing the side-effects of the oral contraceptive pill. Unbeknownst to them, women who went to a family planning clinic were given either the pill or a placebo. The researchers triumphantly proclaimed that side-effects from the pill were no greater than those occurring whilst taking a placebo. The fact that ten women in the 'control group' had ten unwanted pregnancies was deemed an unfortunate and unpreventable consequence of a properly conducted trial. An attempt to conduct a randomised controlled trial on the use of Vitamin B and folic acid as a preventive measure for women who had already had a baby with spina bifida (and therefore had a 1:20 chance of having a second) was stopped as a result of the protests of participating paediatricians.

What woman offered an uncertain but good chance to save her baby from an uncertain but appalling fate, would agree to enter such a trial if she knew the conditions? What does she care about statistical significance and why should she care? In the name of what implacable stony-faced god of numbers is she being asked to sacrifice her child?[12]

The need to ascertain which of two treatments is superior is clearly an important ethical question. If the method used to obtain such knowledge is itself unethical, then the knowledge acquired will almost certainly be only partially valid and not be generalisable to patients as whole people. Put another way: 'If morality and methodology conflict it seems to us that the onus is upon us to develop methodologies that harmonise with our morality rather than compromise with morality on the probably false assumption that we are dealing with an immaculate methodology.'[13]

The moral and ethical issues that surround the conduct of controlled trials is the issue of informed consent. How much is the patient told – indeed is the patient told that she is taking part in a trial, and, if she is told, is she told the whole truth? Informed consent and the issue of paternalism are almost impossible to separate, for the amount of information given to a patient by a doctor is often determined by the doctor's decision as to 'how much the patient needs to know'. It is argued that in the same way as parents may sometimes have to act in the child's best interest against the child's wishes, a doctor may have to act against the patient's wishes or manipulate and distort information in such a way that the patient's best interest (as determined by the doctor) is protected. It is clear that a certain amount of authoritarianism, paternalism and domination may be necessary for the doctor to be effective in the patient's best interest, e.g. when the patient is in an acute medical emergency through, say, shock or loss of consciousness. The question arises whether the doctor transfers this necessary authoritative approach to assess the 'best interests of the patient' in less acute circumstances. Paternalism, or the 'Doctor knows best' attitude has for decades gone unchallenged. The decision whether or not to tell a patient that he has a terminal disease, whether to embark on a particular operation, or proceed with a life-saving procedure, has almost always been determined by doctors, usually on their own. Often this is done because it is judged to be in the patient's best interest, and the patient is judged to be not in a position to make the decision or is unable to make a proper assessment. Where there are decisions concerning whether a severely handicapped child should live or die, doctors have felt it is their responsibility to shoulder the burden. 'In the end it is usually the doctor who has to decide the issue: it is . . . cruel to ask the parents whether they want their child to live or die:[14] This wish to protect the patient is laudable when it arises from altruistic motives, but it is not always clear whether it does not also protect the doctor from sharing and struggling with uncertainty and conflict. The pursuit of an analytic and scientific mode of thinking in problem-solving makes it much more difficult to tolerate the confusion and messiness of complex moral, legal and ethical problems. Indeed it may result in the doctor being peculiarly unqualified in arriving at such decisions.

> Once the complexity of these judgements is appreciated and once their evaluative character is understood, it is impossible to hold that the physician is in a better position to make them than the patient or his family. The failure to ask what sort of harm/benefit judgements may properly be made by the physician in his capacity as a physician is a fundamental feature of medical paternalism.[15]

It is a sad reflection of how far medical thinking has developed and narrowed that one of the leaders of the profession could say 'Most doctors like to believe that medicine is more art than science. That is a dangerous doctrine. If true it means we are little better than quacks and open to the same criticisms'.[16] And another – in relation to informed consent in controlled trials: 'Over my dead body'.[17]

Unless medicine as a discipline can begin to feel secure enough to acknowledge and develop its own philosophical and scientific base, rather than borrow those that belong to other disciplines, it will develop along pathways that lead to a 'tyranny of excellence'[16] that confuses facts with truths and divorces it from the real problems of real people. Or, as Prince Charles more modestly stated: 'The whole imposing edifice of modern medicine for all its breathtaking success is like the celebrated Tower of Pisa, slightly off balance.[18]

5

The Planet Strikes Back

Man's concern with the environment is not new – as long ago as 400 BC, soil erosion concerned Plato and in 900 AD it brought down the Mayan civilisation in Central America. Many so-called 'primitive' tribes in North America and the Far East lived according to the laws of Nature, and were, and still are, appalled by the white man's disregard for the fundamental principles of preservation and conservation. Industrialised society has brought many benefits to mankind but in its trail has left us with a legacy of industrial diseases. The smog in London in 1952 was responsible for 3–4,000 deaths and the Clean Air Bill passed in 1956 was a first step in the politicisation of environmental causes.[1]

The need to care for the environment is the one overriding and unifying belief that binds the Green movement together. The impact of the environment on health is also not a twentieth-century concern. Living in accordance with the laws of Nature was one of Hippocrates' basic principles of good health. This treatise, *De aere, aquis et locis* (On airs, waters and places), suggests that the Green movement, Friends of the Earth, the Ecology Party and other environmental groups may be drawing on very deep concerns that can be identified throughout man's history. These movements are not just the product of an idealistic, anti-authoritarian, 'back to nature' movement with which they are often associated, but articulate for us a point of view which has always been present in man's understanding.

1. Whoever wishes to investigate medicine properly should proceed thus: in the first place to consider the seasons of the year, and what effects each of them produces. . . . Then the winds, the hot and the cold, especially such as are common to all countries, and then such as are peculiar to each locality. We must also consider the qualities. In the same manner, when one

comes into a city to which he is a stranger, he ought to consider its situation, how it lies as to the winds and the rising of the sun; for its influence is not the same whether it lies to the north or the south, to the rising or to the setting sun. These things one ought to consider most attentively, and concerning the waters which the inhabitants use, whether they be marshy and soft, or hard, and running from elevated and rocky situations, and then if saltish and unfit for cooking; and the ground, whether it be naked and deficient in water, or wooded and well watered, and whether it lies in a hollow, confined situation, or is elevated and cold; and the mode in which the inhabitants live, and what are their pursuits, whether they are fond of drinking and eating to excess, and given to indolence, or are fond of exercise and labour, and not given to excess in eating and drinking. [2]

A more recent position regarding man's relationship to his environment and the influence this has on his health is Claude Bernard's famous dictum (*La fixité du milieu intérieur est la condition essentielle de la vie libre* – The constancy of the internal environment is the essential condition of independent life). The phrase '*le milieu intérieur*' has entered medical thinking and, under the influence of W. B. Cannon, it was recognised that this *milieu intérieur* could be kept 'fixed' only if it was in a particular relationship with the *milieu extérieur* (external environment). Cannon developed his ideas to include the theory of homoeostasis – the stability of bodily functions necessitated a balance between internal and external environment. It was however Selye in the 1920s who further expanded Cannon's work and developed our modern understanding of stress and stress disorders. [3] His work has allowed us to understand the connection between psychological factors (unhappiness, anger, despair), physical factors (noise levels, air pollution, humidity) and physiological functioning (blood pressure, circulating hormone levels, immunological competence). Medical science can indeed grasp the significance of the 'balance' between the *milieu intérieur* and the *milieu extérieur* even if medical practice has remained fragmented.

In the last three decades medical practice has been fascinated by the minutiae of medical technology and the concepts expounded by Bernard, Cannon and Selye have made little impact. The problem of the environmental influence on health has thus largely been ignored by medicine. It has been left to the environmentalists and ecologists to point out the links and the dangers.

Several of the seminal books that were written in the Sixties *Limits to Growth*,[4] *Population Bomb*,[5] *Only One Earth*,[6] appeared to portray such a bleak picture and many of their wilder predictions were so patently wrong that for a while their warnings and suggested solutions were ridiculed and disregarded. More recently, there has been a clear and radical shift amongst establishment institutions, food manufacturers, multi-national corporations, politicians and governments. It is possible to say, 'We're all environmentalists now', something that was not even thinkable a few years ago. Whether this change has come soon enough and whether the political will really does exist to ensure the fundamental alterations required are enacted, it is still too early to say, but the climate of opinion in which the debate is taking place has altered, and global solutions are indeed being considered for many of the problems that man, in his rapacious and greedy way, has wrought on the environment.

Before exploring some of these problems in detail, it is important to remember that man is capable of environmental improvements as well and that developments in housing, nutrition, education, sanitation have resulted already in a far greater life expectancy for the average person in the developed countries. Prehistoric man did not live beyond eighteen years. This figure rose to thirty-three in the middle ages and in 1860 it was forty-three and now it is seventy, and seventy-five for women.[7] Even with this clear evidence that man must have done something right in his attempt to improve 'life on earth', it is necessary to ask the question – at what price? There are those who would argue that the improvements and technological advances of the last century have so upset the ecological balance that we are in mortal danger and 'as we sow, so shall we reap'. Thus many of the concerns, diseases and epidemics affecting us today are the direct result of the influence of the environment upon us, and to ignore the consequences any longer is a luxury we can no longer afford.

Physical environment

It is not difficult to look for and find direct relationships between the climatic conditions and health. Indeed numerous authors through the ages have drawn attention to the links: Arbuthnot's

Table 7 Reported effects of the influence of weather and climate on diseases (abridged from Tromp (1963) and assembled by Maunder (1970))

Short periodical effects	*Long periodical effects (seasonal or pseudo-seasonal)*
Lung diseases	
Tuberculosis: Haemoptysis suddenly increases in clinics after oppressive warm weather before thunderstorms, after föhn, humid cold foggy weather or sudden heatwaves	Increased sensitivity to tuberculin test in March and April; low during autumn
Asthma (bronchial): Increases with sudden cooling (particularly if accompanied by falling barometric pressure and rising wind speed); during high barometric pressure and fog (in W. Europe) very low asthma frequency	Low in winter, suddenly increasing after June, max. in late autumn (W. Europe)
Bronchitis: Increasing complaints during fog (particularly in air-polluted areas) and specially if accompanied by atmospheric cooling	High in winter, low in summer (in W. Europe)
Hay fever (and various forms of rhinitis): Allergic reactions often increase during atmospheric cooling	Hay fever is related to flowering of certain plants or grasses, different for different countries. In W. Europe usually max. complaints in May–June
Cancer	—
Skin cancer: More common with increasing number of sun-hours and increased exposure of the skin to the sun	
Rheumatic diseases	
Most forms of arthritis react on strong cooling (falling temp.; strong wind). Humidity seems to have no direct effect, only indirect through cooling	Arthritic complaints particularly common in autumn and early winter (W. Europe)

Heart diseases *Coronary thrombosis,* *Myocardial infarction, and* *Angina pectoris:* Occur more frequently shortly after a period of strong cooling	Highest mortality in Jan–Feb (in W. Europe and northern USA), lowest July–Aug. In hot countries (e.g. southern USA) highest mortality in summer, lowest in winter
Infectious diseases *Common cold:* Weather changes affecting thermoregulation mechanism, membrane permeability, and growth and transmission of common cold virus seem to initiate the diseases (e.g. very cold period followed by sudden warming up)	Max. in Feb–March; increasing from Sept–March (in W. Europe)
Influenza: Rel. humidity below 50 per cent and low wind speeds seem to favour the development and transmission of influenza virus	Max. in Dec–Feb; increasing from Sept–March

An Essay Concerning the Effects of Air on Human Bodies (1733), Huxham's *Observationes de Aere et Morbis Epidemica* (1739) and Clark's *The Influence of Climate in the Prevention and Cure of Chronic Disease* (1830). Table 7 illustrates how some diseases have been linked to climatic conditions. It is not only the scientists who were aware of this link. Many of the healing and spiritual centres, built in different cultures across the world, were built on specially chosen sites where climatic conditions were thought to be most favourable. The ancient art of Geomancy was an attempt to understand how the effects of light, sound and water, heat and magnetic radiation influenced man. Like astrology and alchemy, 'ancient sciences' have been abandoned and devalued. Increasingly, however, we are having to return to the question they attempted to address, and re-evaluate their methods and develop new approaches. Our own subjective experience has led us to identify qualities associated with specific regions which can be labelled very bracing, bracing, average, relaxing and very relaxing. Similarly the centre of cities, certain office buildings and high-rise flats are felt to be unhealthy and damaging. The factors which add up to our physical environment and objectively and subjectively lead to these observations are still not fully understood but some attempts to clarify them have been undertaken and the most important ones include:

Air pollution   The dramatic improvement that occurred in English cities following the introduction of smoke-free zones in cities and the Clean Air Act illustrate that change is possible where there is political will. In the course of five days in December 1952 'the great smog' caused the deaths of between 3,000 and 4,000 persons from chronic bronchitis in London alone. The 'smog' was a mixture of fog, smoke and sulphur dioxide particles. The average concentration of sulphur dioxide in urban areas is about 200 microgrammes per cubic metre but during the worst of the smog, the concentration rose to between 7,000 and 8,000 microgrammes. Following the Clean Air Act, London's average duration of bright sunshine rose by 44 minutes a day and Glasgow's by 20 minutes. Further legislation has been enacted to address the problems created by more recent pollutants – smoke from cigarettes, lead from car exhausts, CFCs from aerosol sprays and radiation from the nuclear industry.

Lead   Every year over 2,500 tonnes of lead are released through car exhausts into the earth's atmosphere. It is only within the last ten years that the problem has been recognised. Sweden first introduced unleaded petrol in 1985 and, within a year, 67 per cent of cars able to take unleaded petrol were doing so. In Britain 50 per cent of all petrol stations now serve unleaded petrol and 25 per cent of car owners use it. The health hazard identified although never conclusively proved was the link between lead atmospheric pollution and brain damage, especially in young children.[8]

   Lead poisoning following an acute ingestion will produce symptoms of nausea, headache, loss of appetite, fatigue and irritability. More serious long-term effects include anaemia, kidney damage, nervous system disorders and impaired intellectual functioning. Much of this has been known to medical science for decades. It is the effect of low-level exposure that has only recently become recognised as a health hazard. Tap water samples from the homes of men with high blood pressure have shown consistently higher levels of lead than those homes of men with normal blood pressure. The use of lead-based exterior paint for bridges and other steel structures has resulted in the soil content below such structures containing 48 times more lead than normal. Children living next to such areas were found to have increased amounts of lead in their blood.[9]

CFCs and the ozone layer The ozone layer is a thin layer of an unstable form of oxygen found in the stratosphere. Twelve miles high, it is now known to absorb ultraviolet solar radiation. The latter is known to cause skin cancer and the destruction of the ozone layer has resulted in, amongst other things, a rise in skin cancer. Chlorofluorocarbons (CFCs) are used as a propellant fluid in many aerosols, cans, refrigerants and solvents. Each chlorine molecule found in CFCs can destroy 100,000 molecules of ozone and the discovery of seasonal 'holes' in the ozone layer have now been reported in both the Arctic and Antarctic polar caps. The US Government banned the use of CFCs in 1978, but the UK was still producing 600 million aerosol cans a year containing CFCs as late as 1987. However, by the end of 1989, 85 per cent of all aerosol cans produced were free of CFCs. CFCs can last for more than a hundred years in the atmosphere and it will be many years before we know whether the co-ordinated action taken by the US and the European Community has reversed the damage already done.[10]

Sunlight The lack of sunlight in winter has been identified as a causative factor in some people with depression – the winter blues. This condition, now relabelled SAD (seasonal affective disorder) received scientific respectability when it was identified that light suppresses the hormone melatonin which is produced in greater quantities during winter. SAD sufferers find their symptoms respond to changes in climate and latitude and, more recently, light therapy has been introduced for the treatment of depression.

Sick building syndrome Through the use of health diaries and daily symptom reporting, certain clusters of non-specific complaints (lethargy, tiredness, stuffy nose, headaches) have been identified as being associated with working in particular office buildings. Suggested possible factors include the air-conditioning facilities, the glare from VDUs (visual display units) as well as the level of ionisation. No one factor has been identified and lack of privacy and lack of control of the environment may be equally important elements. The important link, however, is that working in some buildings appears to generate a higher level of unwellness than working in others. Families in high-rise flats *feel* the isolation to a degree that influences their health and wellbeing.

Nuclear radiation   The geopolitical changes that have occurred in the last year and were started with Mikael Gorbachov's rise to power in the USSR will have and have had a great impact on the nuclear industry. The major debates regarding nuclear power as a source of energy for the twenty-first century have had to take on board the profound shifts in the disarmament negotiations currently taking place. For one of the major criticisms levelled against the use of nuclear power as a form of energy was that its production ensured that it was linked to the use of nuclear power as the basis for warfare. Once the link is broken, then the nuclear industry has to justify itself within an increasingly sceptical market economy. Until and unless the problem of disposal of nuclear waste is resolved, and the safety issues surrounding nuclear power stations addressed satisfactorily, the cost of nuclear energy is clearly prohibitive (65 per cent more than coal-fired power and 25 per cent more than oil-fired power), and we are likely to see a return to fossil fuel and alternative sources of energy. In the meantime we are having to respond to the problems of nuclear radiation, the risk of melt-downs, the disposal of nuclear waste and the possibilities of human error. 'The awesome roar which warned of Doomsday' was how one witness described an atomic explosion. The atom bombs dropped on Hiroshima and Nagasaki killed 130,000 and 70,000 people respectively. Until recently, the US and USSR had enough explosive power between them to unleash 1.5 million Hiroshimas. A nuclear bomb that can be stored under a bed has more explosive power than all the explosives used in the Second World War. In 1982, the British Medical Association produced a report on the medical effects of nuclear war in Britain. Its conclusions were that given the predicted level of destruction, no possible medical planning would be of any help.

The problem of waste disposal in the nuclear industry has posed a continuous threat to health and in July 1984 the British Government published a report indicating that the evidence of leukaemia around the Sellafield nuclear plant was one of the highest in the UK. No direct proof could be found that the link was causative, i.e. increased levels of radiation caused leukaemia, but the report raised yet again the concern over the adequacy of controls over discharges from nuclear plants. An earlier report (*Report of the Royal Commission on Environmental Pollution* 1972 chaired by Sir Eric Ashby) had highlighted the dangers without obfuscating the issue. 'In effect we are consciously and deliberately accumulating a toxic substance on the off-chance that it may be possible to get rid of it at a later date. We are committing future generations to tackle the problems which we do not know how to handle.' The problem of pollution is not by any means limited to the nuclear industry. The health hazards resulting from man's indiscriminate abuse of natural resources and criminal disregard for the waste products resulting from this abuse have led to an escalation of the problem which now exists. They can be seen as a combination of environmental degeneration, resources scarcity and a food and water crisis.[11]

Environmental degeneration   To list the ways we have over the centuries polluted our rivers, destroyed our wild life and rendered many other species extinct is both depressing and painful. DDT (used widely as a pesticide for the control of malaria) has been found in polar bears at the North Pole and in penguins at the South Pole. Astronauts on the moon were able to detect the Los Angeles smoke pall from thousands of miles above the earth. The list is endless. Thirty-five per cent of our sewage waste is dumped into the North Sea and has begun to affect quite dramatically the patterns of diseases found in fish. Figure 6 illustrates what was

Figure 6 Pesticides, their uses and the location of residues

Type of pesticide	Uses	Residues occur
Organochlorine	Domestic uses – flysprays, etc.	Foodstuffs – meat, milk, butter, vegetables, fruit
	Infestation control in food stores	
	Animal treatments	Wildlife – insects, worms, birds, predators
Organophosphorus	Agricultural crop spraying	
Herbicides	Seed dressings	Fish and water birds
Fungicides		Waters

Source: Abbott and Thomson (1968).

known in 1968 of the link between pesticides and the food chain. Today's list would be far greater and would have to include the problem of acid rain, deforestation and the greenhouse effect.

Acid rain   Sulphur dioxide and nitrogen emission, principally from the burning of coal and oil are released into the atmosphere in ever-increasing amounts. Some of the sulphur and nitrogen is absorbed into vegetation, but the majority mixes with moisture in the atmosphere and is converted to sulphuric and nitric acid. Rain is naturally acid through carbonic acid pH.5.6. Rain now falling over parts of Europe and North America has a pH of between 4.0 and 5.0. This increased acidity affects lakes, fishes, rivers, soils and plant life. Fish have died in half the lakes in the Canadian province of Ontario. In Poland, railway tracks have been so corroded through acid rain that trains cannot travel at more than 25 mph. Acid rain may be cutting crop yields in Britain by as much as 10 per cent, costing British farmers £200 million a year.[12]

Deforestation   The destruction of forests has increased the risk of soil erosion through rain and floods. Shelter provided for wild life is decreased and the recycling of oxygen and absorption of carbon dioxide is diminished. It is estimated that nearly 29 million acres of forest are destroyed annually – some of it for timber and paper production – the remainder so that the land can be used for agriculture, mostly the raising of beef cattle, an uneconomical use of resources. Conversion to cattle-ranching results in what has been called the 'hamburger connection', for nearly all the beef produced by six Central American countries is exported to the United States. The average European uses 265 lbs of paper and board a year, whilst the figure for the average Indian is 4.4 lbs. The effect of losing so much of the world's natural resources is not fully understood, but the predominant concern is the effect on levels of carbon dioxide in the atmosphere and the consequent changes in global warming.[13]

Greenhouse effect   As a result of burning fossil fuels, carbon dioxide is released into the atmosphere. In addition, with the reduction of natural forests, the amount of carbon dioxide absorbed back into the vegetation is reduced. It is estimated that the atmosphere contains 15–20 per cent more carbon dioxide than it did in 1850 and that if we were to continue our present level of combustion this figure would double in forty-five years. The heat from the sun's rays are either absorbed in the atmosphere (10 –20%), reflected back to space (35–50%) or reach the surface of the earth (45–50%). As the level of carbon dioxide in the atmosphere rises, the amount of solar radiation reflected back into space falls. The long-term result has been a gradual increase in the earth's temperature – the best accepted estimate is that a doubling of carbon dioxide increases the earth's temperature by 2°–3°C. The effect of this rise is unpredictable but one has to remember that it took a 4° rise to bring the earth out of its last Ice Age 10,000 years ago. A further rise would inevitably have an effect on wind, rainfall, ocean circulation patterns and the Polar ice caps. Although the direct effect on health is not immediately obvious – the rise in atmospheric temperature could disrupt the ecosystem, interfere with life-cycles and influence the world's crop-growing regions. It is not necessary to prove a *direct causal* link – but to remember the *connectedness* between one aspect or the environment – the temperature – and other features.[14]

Resource scarcity   A major concern of present times is whether or not supplies of sources of energy will be adequate in the future. At present 96 per cent of all our energy needs are supplied through fossil fuels (coal, oil, natural gas). Estimates in the late Seventies suggested that, on present trends, oil and natural gas would last another fifty years and coal another hundred and fifty. Energy consumption has trebled since 1945 and it is estimated to double again by the year 2000. In the last few years there has been evidence to suggest that oil consumption is dropping in the prosperous Northern hemisphere but it is still true that the average consumption of energy in the prosperous North is fifteen times that of someone in the Southern hemisphere. Attempts to develop alternative forms of energy – wind power, solar heat, and the use of ethyl-alcohol in motor cars – are still fairly isolated but at some stage governments will have to wake up to the fact that the world's resources are finite and dwindling fast.

Kenneth Boulding has said anyone who believes exponential growth can go on forever in a finite world is either a madman or an economist. The Earth cannot much longer support what he has called the 'cowboy economy' of the past, the reckless exploitative behaviour of men facing what seemed an open frontier of unlimited riches. Instead we shall need a 'spaceman economy' in which we do not maximise production and consumption as 'income' but respect and conserve the planet's limited resources as 'capital'.[15]

It is quite understandable that when faced with these global descriptions of the problems individuals will feel both distanced by the massive scale of the difficulties and find difficulty in identifying themselves with both the cause of the problem as well as the solution. It is not until the difficulties begin to impinge more directly on individuals that the problems are both recognised and more importantly politicised. This has become increasingly evident over the crisis regarding both food and water consumption.

Food facts

For many in the prosperous North, the food debate often centres on a particular ingredient in our daily diet. Is the level of fibre sufficient? Does the cholesterol content surpass the accepted limit? Should I take supplemental vitamins and minerals? Placed against the background of the problem of malnutrition, famine and starvation in the South these problems appear obscene. On the one hand there exists a multi-million pound slimming industry whilst on the other a third of the world's population go hungry. The US uses as much fertiliser on its lawns and golf courses as India requires to sustain its population with food. The North consumes double the amount of protein per person than the South and derives over 60 per cent of that protein from meat, whereas between 70 and 85 per cent of protein source is derived from vegetables in the South.[16] When taken alongside the fact that meat requires ten times the amount of energy to produce the same quantity of protein as that derived from vegetables, it becomes clear that the problems of the North with its overconsumption and undernutrition are linked to the problems of the South with its underconsumption and subsequent malnutrition.

For the most part, however, the North has focused on the effects of individual diets and patterns of nutrition as specific causative factors in the development of disease. The major epidemics of the last thirty years, coronary heart disease, cancer and degenerative arthritic disease, have all been linked in some form or another to dietary factors. Examining patterns of eating since the Second World War would reveal an 80 per cent increase in the consumption of soft drinks, a 70 per cent increase in consumption of potato crisps. At the same time there has been a 25 per cent decrease in the consumption of dairy products, fruit and vegetables. The proportion of carbohydrate derived from simple sugars has risen from 32 per cent in 1960 to 53 per cent in 1979.[17] The link between optimum health and optimum nutrition has been consistently made throughout the last twenty years. Some of these links are based on good medical facts, others on fanciful conjecture. The link between low levels of dietary fibre and such diverse disease predominantly found in developed countries, e.g. gall bladder disease, diverticulitis, haemorrhoids and colonic cancer, is now well-established, whereas the widespread use of supplemental vitamin C in 'boosting resistance' is not.[18] The preoccupation of many middle-class people – the worried well – with perfection and longevity has mushroomed into a preoccupation with the minutiae of diet that has led several authorities to condemn this preoccupation as a form of obsession not dissimilar to anorexia nervosa and other eating disorders.

Nevertheless, the constant attention food receives in the media, especially women's magazines, has ensured the debate regarding food would sooner or later spill over into the political arena. At first, the battle lines seemed to be drawn over the issue of additives in food – not without just concern. At present over half the additives found in food are there for aesthetic or commercial reasons. The average adult is said to consume the equivalent of twenty-two aspirin-sized tablets of additives a day.[19] An increasing and impressive array of statistics and reports draws attention to the potential health hazards and the incidence of food intolerance and food allergies suggested that we were witnessing a new epidemic. Medical opinion was divided and many of the claims made by practitioners of a new specialty – clinical ecology – were disregarded and devalued by the orthodox establishment.[20] Nevertheless, the links between the increasing use of additives and so-called 'food allergies' has become so strong that legislation forcing manufacturers to identify all additives on food packaging was introduced and the guide to additives, *E for Additives*, became a bestseller.[21] However, it was with the salmonella scare in 1988–89 that 'healthy food' entered the political centre stage, leading to the resignation of Edwina Currie as Health Minister. Her remarks regarding the contamination of eggs with salmonella produced a drop in sales that required a major government subsidy to poultry farmers and the establishment of a separate agency to ensure that the links between the agricultural lobby and the 'healthy food' lobby were strengthened. The public is now increasingly sophisticated regarding the 'right' and 'wrong' sorts of food. Consumer pressure has ensured that all major supermarket stores now have 'health food' sections and have rapidly espoused the cause of Green consumerism and ecologically friendly products. Whether these changes will have a lasting effect on agricultural policy and food consumption is too early to say, but it is clear that awareness of the link between food and health has risen to the level that no government can ignore this area of policy.

The concern over healthy food was supported by the increasing concern over the purity of our drinking water.

Water

It would be difficult to imagine that ten years ago debates regarding the purity of drinking water would become national news, yet concern regarding the scarcity of water as a resource and the effect of pollution on wild life, fish and the human species have been present for decades, if not centuries. Water has always affected our health, be it as a source of infection as a result of pollution – the great epidemics of typhoid, cholera and dysentery are all water-borne infections, or as a source of healing and cleanliness. The mineralised waters of Vichy, Bath, Baden-Baden and other well-known spas have long been associated with recuperation and convalescence – 'taking the waters' was a common nineteenth-century remedy and several of the sacred healing sites reputed to have miraculous healing powers were found over deep wells or next to running 'pure' water.[22]

'Pure' water has always symbolised cleanliness and health but such is the demand for the use of water that purification plants re-use water many times before it is discarded through sewage. For years this process was thought to be quite safe and the major water-borne infections of the nineteenth century were viewed with only historical interest by community physicians and public health managers. Not only did the problem of water scarcity begin to reappear but new water-borne infections and impurities were identified in tap drinking-water, leading the European Commission to penalise the UK for having lower levels of safety than were permissible to Common Market policy. The major concern is focused on the level of nitrates in tap water which has been steadily increasing over the last two decades and now exceeds the acceptable limit in certain parts of the country. Nitrates in the water result from artificial fertilisers, domestic sewage effluent and slurry from intensive livestock units. Again the health link is tenuous but high levels of nitrate ingestion have been linked with certain forms of cancer. At present, at least sixteen toxic pesticides can be identified in drinking water and there is no accepted policy regarding testing and decontamination.[23] As water consumption increased the problem began to mount and the recent privatisation of water supplies has done little to reassure the public that the problems will be addressed. We may need to wait for another Chadwick (1800–1890), author of the *Report on the Sanitary Conditions of the Labouring Population of Great Britain* (1842) which formed the basis of the nineteenth-century public health legislation and from which we derive much of the health benefits of the twentieth century, before further changes are introduced.

It is increasingly clear that if we are to understand the relationship between ill-health and ecological destabilisation the medical profession will need to involve itself more directly in matters regarding the environment. Not only are many of the modern epidemics (heart disease, arthritis, cancer) partly related to environmental factors but political reaction stimulated by the rise of the Green movement will ensure that no government will be able to ignore the validity of public concern. The specialties of community health, environmental health and occupational health have all been relegated to Cinderella status in the medical profession. The next two decades may see these areas of medicine encouraging more government research than the 'high status' specialties of heart surgery, transplantation and genetic engineering.

However, it will be important for medical researchers to understand the difference between a science that looks for *causes* and a science that looks for *connections*. We can only begin to grasp the message that underpins the greening process if we recognise the need to broaden the accepted definition of science and the scientific method.

6

The Patient Wakes Up

> I was aware in the next minute after this refusal to change his
> tablets that he was probably going to attack me if I persisted.
> I remember thinking 'Well at least it will be interesting' – he
> grabbed me by the collar saying he was going to fucking kill
> me, that all doctors were the same. They'd done this to him
> to begin with and now they just treated him like a little kid.
> He let go of me and began to cry. I gave him a prescription
> and 'phoned the psychiatrist. Later I cried too – a mixture of
> shakiness, fear and melodramatic exhilaration.[1]

This graphic illustration of an encounter between doctor and
patient highlights the issue of power and control in a most
dramatic way. For a few moments the patient attempts to summon
up his repressed urge for control and challenges not only the
doctor himself but the whole profession of medicine. If he had
succeeded in 'fucking killing the doctor' he would have been faced
with the full authority of the professions of law and religion. Issues
of power and control are played out in almost every consultation,
whether it is a decision to give a prescription, withhold information, provide a certificate to legitimise absence from work or
sign a medical examination form that permits a seventy-five-year-
old to continue to hold a car licence. Increasingly, decisions
regarding the prolongation of life, the termination of pregnancy or
the appropriateness of heroic surgery have begun to impinge on
the freedom of the doctor to be in control. Research trials with
complex and often dangerous drugs require informed consent
where patients are expected to give their permission. The introduction of computers into medical settings has highlighted the
problem of confidentiality of medical notes and underlined the
concern as to what exactly is written in the notes. The rise of
consumerism, one of the main features of the Green movement,

has meant that patients are increasingly challenging, either individually or through their representative organisations, the monopoly of power the medical profession has appeared to maintain over health issues.

Gods, doctors and mortals

The primordial healer or shaman owed his power to the demi-world in which he lived – that between the Gods and man. Aesculapius, Hermes and Chiron, Greek figures linked to healing, were all half-God half-man. Arab and Jewish physicians were less closely connected to the priesthood though many of the mediaeval European physicians maintained a link with matters 'supernatural' through their study of alchemy. Whether or not doctors were closely associated with the church, they were seen as powerful figures through their knowledge and/or contact with the Gods. The need to be powerful was inherent in their work. When a healthy man develops an illness and becomes a patient, his responses shift from adult to child: he becomes dependent on those around him and seeks comfort and care. His ability to care for his own body is diminished and he seeks the help of powerful others. This regression to a dependent state may be a necessary prelude to recovery; however, those who cannot allow themselves to regress and be cared for when they become ill may do so for fear of losing control.

In time of illness, the doctor is seen as someone who with his knowledge and expertise will restore the patient's ability to regain control of his body or mind. It is because so much power is invested in him by the patient that the doctor or healer needs to be aware of his own powerlessness. The forming metaphor or archetype for the shaman-healer, doctor-priest, therapist-counsellor has been that of the wounded healer. Chiron, the centaur, was entrusted with Aesculapius as a young boy. It was from him that Aesculapius learnt his medical skills. Yet Chiron had an incurable wound. Many a doctor has witnessed how his understanding and skills are enhanced if he himself experiences an illness. In the course of their studies, medical students often 'develop' the illness they are currently studying. They develop the symptoms of multiple sclerosis when first meeting a patient with this complaint. A cough that lasts more than a week is thought to be the first sign of tuberculosis. The headache that does not respond to aspirin is the undiagnosed brain tumour. These internal experiences of 'illness' are a very necessary process of experiencing 'wounds' without actually being wounded. It allows the medical student to go through the modern equivalent of a shamanistic training where he acknowledges his potential for being a patient as well as being a doctor. It is unfortunate that for the majority, these experiences are regarded as being 'neurotic' and the student is encouraged to dismiss them as signs of weakness, so that as he matures he adopts the mantle of only one half of the archetype: that of the healer/doctor with little or no perception of the opposite pole. This opposite pole is then projected on to the patient so that feelings of weakness, dependency and helplessness are avoided by the doctor. Projection is that process by which we first 'repress' and then cast out those aspects of ourselves which we do not like or cannot accept. Someone who sees himself as 'good' will see 'evil' around him. The husband who sees himself as rational, intellectual and clear will berate his wife for being irrational, emotional and muddled. The process of separating the good and bad aspects of ourselves and only accepting or being conscious of one side of ourselves is a psychological process which psycho-analysts refer to as 'splitting'.

It is this 'splitting' of the archetype, or inborn potential, of the 'wounded healer' that helps to produce the one-sided power relationships between doctors and patients. All the wounds are lodged in the patient and all the healing is attributed to the doctor. The coming together of the powerful doctor and the wounded patient allows for an external union to occur.

The rise and fall of the professional

The doctor needs his patients just as much as the patient needs his doctor. When this process of projecting the unwanted or unconscious attribute is organised and institutionalised, we begin to see the development of the professional doctor and the professional patient, each keeping to and obeying rules of conduct determined by the need to identify with one pole of the archetype. Thus someone experiencing an illness may be required to adopt the 'sick role' in order to receive medical help. This 'sick role', as described by Parsons,[2] has four components. The patient will be exempted from responsibility for his illness and be allowed to withdraw from his social and work obligations, only if he accepts the help and medicine given to him by his doctor and only if he makes every effort to improve and get well. A patient who attempts to avoid one or other of these components will find that he will no longer be accepted as a patient, as he has stepped outside the rules laid down by both doctors and patients for an appropriate exchange.

> The professionalism of medicine is directly related to its mono-polisation of 'official' definitions of illness and health. The doctor's certificate defines and legitimates the withdrawal of labour[3]

With the development of medicine as the 'noble profession', doctors took on the role of the 'honoured practitioner'. It was not until the late nineteenth and early part of the twentieth century that the social distance between doctor and patient became accentuated. As the knowledge base and technical skill required to practise medicine grew, the doctor took on the role of the shaman: mysterious, powerful and frightening. He was accorded privileges that were special to his status. He could park his car wherever he liked, have his telephone repaired urgently, avoid jury duty etc. A Marxist analysis of the profession of medicine might draw attention to the role of power in the medical division of labour, and note how the medical monopoly ensures the subser-vience of other para-medical groups. The control exercised by the medical profession has been described in similar terms to the professions of law and religion as the method by which control is exercised on behalf of the State to ensure a suppressed, ignorant and subservient working class.[4]

Feminist sociologists have drawn attention to the male-dominated patriarchal society within most Western cultures in which the medical profession with its emphasis on male values of effort, control and suppression contributes to the established order. Central to this critique is the male-orientated view of the management of female sexuality and reproduction which has given rise to numerous recent attacks on the medical profession.[5] To some extent these views are supported in studies of doctors and medical students.

For example, the intake of medical students is still predomi-nantly from the professional middle classes and it is only recently that women have been accorded parity in the places offered to students. Questionnaire surveys of medical students suggest that they exhibit many of the characteristics of the authoritarian personality (they identify with established social order, are resistant to change, dislike uncertainty, accept dictates of authority). This, coupled with the overtly male culture associated with medical schools, lends weight to the critiques offered by both Marxists and feminists.

Once established, the professions ensure that their control over their particular area of expertise maintains their occupational monopoly. First, they determine who can or cannot enter the profession. Methods are developed for expelling a member who has transgressed the accepted code of conduct. Secondly, they endeavour to maintain a clientèle that is dependent on the services that only they are able to provide. They alone have the knowledge and, often the legal protection to provide those services. Thirdly, they attempt to protect their special status and privilege by ensuring their autonomy and right to determine their own methods of accountability. A more benign view of the profession of medicine would stress the importance of a number of attributes: the acquisition of theoretical knowledge and skill base; the development of specialised educational centres; the examination and testing of competence of individual members, and the development of a professional code of conduct and ethical standards. The same view might underline the importance of social altruism, professional competence, social responsibility and service to the client. For many within the profession of medicine, financial transactions and a business orientation would be viewed as counter to the ethic of a professional person.

The professions, including medicine, have experienced serious erosions of their status over the last ten to fifteen years. A number of different factors have contributed to this process not least the decentralising or proletarianisation of knowledge and power. Proletarianisation has been defined as a process involving 1) the worker performing a limited number of tasks, 2) the worker having little or no say in his conditions of work (hours, character of work, tasks to be performed), 3) the worker being on a salaried wage and limited in any further earnings he may accrue, and 4) the worker attaching himself to a collective organisation (trade union) in order to protect himself from exploitation.[6] In the context of the 'greening process' such influences in medicine can be interpreted as a consequence of the knowledge revolution, the self-help and consumer movement, the rise of the 'ancillary' medical professions, especially nursing and midwifery, and including the 'alternative' professions of chiropractic, osteopathy etc. Additionally, the development of bureaucracy in medical care has eroded the directness of the relationship between the professional and his client. The rise of the intermediary through the hospital administrator, the health economist and the civil servant in the Department of Health has introduced a third force which challenges and undermines the prerogative of the professional in the determination of working hours and financial rewards. In the light of these factors it becomes increasingly clear that medicine, once the 'noble profession', has in its attempt to adapt to forces within society, found itself moving away from its traditional professional base to one where it is seen as operating as a trade union.

Knowledge explosion and the right to know

A physician's ability to preserve his own power over the patient in the doctor–patient relationship depends largely on his ability to control the patient's uncertainty. The physician enhances his power to the extent that he can maintain the patient's uncertainty about the course of illness, efficacy of therapy or specific future actions of the physician himself.[7]

That knowledge is power is an axiom as true in medicine as in any other aspect of our lives. Whilst the balance of knowledge is heavily weighted against the patient, it is very difficult for the individual to feel secure enough to challenge the professional or indeed to believe that he has a right to know. The change amongst the public, however, appears unstoppable: newspaper articles, magazines, television programmes, self-help books have increased the availability and accessibility of this knowledge base. Initially such sources were ascribed to eminent medical personnel signing themselves 'Dr Harley' or 'Dr Wimpole'. The breaking down of the barriers, however, has meant that agony aunts, professional journalists and social activists have been able to provide information directly to the public in a way that challenges the knowledge monopoly of the medical profession. The natural-birth movement, critics of Caesarean section, hysterectomies, tonsillectomies, indiscriminate tranquilliser use, radical mastectomies, all found their advocates in the increasingly knowledgeable lay middle-class. In 1975 the Boston Women's health book

Our Bodies, Ourselves became a symbol of the decade that was to herald the knowledge explosion.[8] Women were taught by other non-medical women how to practise birth control, regulate their periods, manage their menopausal symptoms and examine their cervix.

Discrepant attitudes on the right to know about one's illness are no better illustrated than in the area of cancer and terminal illness. Numerous surveys indicate that the great majority of patients wish to know the truth about their condition whilst a disproportionate number of doctors feel that the patient should be protected from the truth.[9] This paternalistic attitude amongst doctors has been shown increasingly to reflect their own difficulties and inabilities to handle the emotional consequences of 'truth telling'. Courses in 'breaking bad news' for doctors, although helping to provide some guidance, generally have failed to cope with the defensiveness of the profession. Increasingly, nurse-counsellors and psychologists have been introduced into medical settings to allow for the 'truth telling' process to be adequately monitored. As doctors allow themselves to be marginalised, so they begin to lose some of their power. Several other areas of medicine have seen the introduction of consumer rights. Ethical considerations involving transplant surgery, abortion, in-vitro fertilisation, the prolongation of life in heart-lung machines have been witness to the realisation that doctors are no better and no worse at making these decisions than other informed members of the public.

As the doctor's sole prerogative over these life and death issues is challenged, so his power-base becomes weaker. In the area of research and clinical trials, the nature of informed consent has become a central issue and the patient's moral, legal and ethical rights are seen as being undermined by the sole prerogative that the medical profession has over the conduct of such trials.[10] Five principles of *autonomy* (the individual's freedom to decide), *veracity* (truthfulness), *justice* (equal though different contribution from both doctor and patient), *beneficence* (the duty to do good) and *non-malfeasance* (positive principle not to do harm) have been suggested as the basis to an agreed 'Bill of Rights'.[11] The movement in the recognition of the needs for such a Bill is an extension of the human rights movement of the sixties where emphasis was placed on civil, racial and sexual non-discrimination. The Helsinki Agreement in 1975,[12] together with the Nuremberg

Code on medical experimentation,[13] has laid down guidelines which accord patients protection against unethical experimentation. Charters on the Rights of Patients have now been passed by both the American Hospital Association[14] as well as the European Parliament.[15] These legal moves determined by State and parliamentary legislation supersede the Hippocratic oath which for many years stood as the primary code of conduct defined by doctors for doctors. Both the public and the State now recognise that the medical profession cannot be allowed to provide its own code of conduct. The result of this has been the gradual introduction of constraints and responsibilities on the individual doctor which erode his traditional power-base and sense of autonomy.

Doctors and other health-care professionals

At the same time as the patient has 'woken up' and demanded his rights, doctors have had to face the challenge to their authority from other health-care professionals who have traditionally assumed a subordinate and subservient role towards doctors. The medical profession has ensured its position as the dominant profession in health-care by exercising both educational and legislative control over other professions. In addition, it commands obedience amongst its own members by ensuring that the hierarchy and authority of the individual doctor is protected by threat of disciplinary procedure.

The Council (General Medical) recognises and welcomes the growing contribution made to health-care by nurses and other persons who have been trained to perform specialised functions . . . [but] the doctor should retain ultimate responsibility for the management of his patients because only the doctor has received the necessary training to undertake this responsibility.

For this reason a doctor who improperly delegates to a person who is not a registered medical practitioner functions requiring the knowledge and skill of a medical practitioner is liable to disciplinary procedures.[16]

This attempt to legislate to protect medical dominance and to ensure professional and occupational subordination has been increasingly challenged by the 'subordinate' professions which include nursing, midwifery, pharmacy, dentistry, optometry and, more recently, members of the so-called alternative professions – chiropractic, osteopathy, acupuncture etc.

The nursing profession has a long and well-established link with the medical profession. It is still predominantly a female profession and the role of nurse as the mother/wife/servant to the father/husband/master (doctor) still forms the basis to the working relationship that can be observed in most clinical settings. The word 'nurse' with its connotation of mothering and suckling reflects the traditional role of nursing babies and the sick, while the nurse is seen as the substitute mother looking after the 'baby'/patient, and while the 'father'/doctor instructs and controls the family. Ironically, it was Florence Nightingale who gave rise to the model of the nurse as the organised housewife, the caring mother and the obedient servant – exemplifying the virtues of the Victorian upper-middle-class woman. Although nursing as a profession has always been separated from the religious orders it has nevertheless failed to gain the autonomy necessary to ensure its own independent professional status. Features of the nursing profession such as low pay, low prestige, unsocial hours, lack of job autonomy, and high turnover of personnel have ensured that it retains its dependent relationship with the medical profession. Nurses have been traditionally accorded separate privileges to compensate for this low status. In the past they were referred to either as 'Angels of Mercy (Madonna)', or sexual fantasy objects (whores) with the power issues between doctors and nurses often revolving around a hidden and usually unspoken sexual game. The nature of this 'game' was increasingly exposed as nurses themselves became aware of its exploitive nature. Sociological studies have drawn attention to the underlying assumptions that underpin the nursing role, i.e. that of mothering, and likening the hospital ward to the home situation. As a result, nurses have begun to free themselves from a role-model that has previously maintained their subservience to the doctor. The duty to follow the doctor's instructions at all times, even when the nurse knew that the patient's life was endangered, has been replaced by an increasing refusal to obey silently. As nurses have demanded more autonomy and independence they have emphasised the independent contribution and the importance of the 'nursing process'. 'Nurses are near the patients around the clock and yet they have the least formal responsibility compared with attending physicians or house-staff.'[17]

At the same time nurses began to challenge their own teachers and question the relevance of the training they were receiving. Student nurses

. . . could detect little meaning in their daily work patterns. Many of them found it impossible to get explanations of what they were supposed to be doing at all. These difficulties seemed to be ill-understood by those in charge of them, who sought to explain their local difficulties of ward staffing by a decline in the quality of recruits. The survey revealed deep conflicts between the ward sisters and the hospital training staff.[18]

These deep conflicts within the nursing profession have led to several changes which as yet have not had time to establish themselves. 'Project 2000', which has dramatically altered the training offered to nurses, has attempted to give them a college and university base to their education, with academic career structures similar to medicine.[19] The Cumberledge Report recommended the establishment of an independent nurse-practitioner, operating from a separate base to the general practitioner.[20] She would have freedom to provide health-care services including the prescribing of a limited list of drugs to patients who could seek her help directly and need not have a referral letter from the doctor. This direct challenge to the doctor's authority and prerogative has understandably met with much resistance from the medical profession. However, similar challenges have surfaced from opticians, who wish to provide services direct to patients, midwives and pharmacists. The hegemony for so long maintained by the medical profession will not be able to withstand this pressure, especially at a time that the State itself, through Parliament and the Department of Health, is eroding the ability of individual doctors to determine their own work routine.

It is important not to assume that these changes will inevitably benefit the patient or provide a 'better service'. It could be argued that an 'academic' nursing training will drive nurses even further from their vocational ideals. No one can deny that patients when ill and distressed need and require the attention, amongst other things, of a 'good mother'. If nurses are to eschew the roles they have traditionally undertaken, who will there be to provide the comfort and care for patients? The challenge to doctors' authority may indeed be a necessary and an inevitable consequence of changes in our society, but the fragmentation of the 'team' and at times anarchic results may be part of the price that may have to be paid.

The emergence of the team

The bureaucratisation of medicine has led to a further erosion of the doctor's authority with the introduction of the hospital manager and health-care administrator. The impact this has had on the practice of medicine is detailed in a subsequent chapter, but together with the changes in nursing policy and consumer involvement, the once 'tidy' model of medical decision-making is now fragmented and in a state of chaos. Attempts to replace the old hierarchical model with the doctor as the ultimate authority with a new model have focused on the concept of the 'team'.

A review of the literature concerning team-work within health care comprises a litany of disappointment and frustration at the patchiness, or at times the absence, of fruitful and democratic communication between the professionals. The difficulties which are experienced, particularly by the district nurses, health visitors and social workers, are profound and dispiriting.[21] Moreover these difficulties too often result in a failure to provide a good service to the patients.[22] It is symbolic of the nature of the problem that the patient is rarely mentioned in the literature; so great is the level of frustration between the professions that research focuses almost entirely on the identification of the blocks to good communication.

Training for collaboration

The concept of interprofessional collaboration is not something that any of the professions were, or to a great extent are, trained for. If any articulated model of team-work exists within health-care training, it is perhaps that of the operating-theatre team or the 'ward round' team. But here the models are centred on a relatively clearly defined task, ritual roles and a clearly defined hierarchy. The network of communication is in fact a chain of command.

Moreover the operating-theatre model and the 'ward round' model are both centred on the construct of an inert and inactive patient. They both deal with a finite task, the completion of the operation and/or medical care and the discharge of the patient.

Patients with a slow degenerative disease, living within the community, are not inert. They have not been silenced by the technology or the institutionalised rituals of the hospital regime. Their day-to-day lives are situated within a dynamically shifting field of community life. The task of the primary health-care team is not finite in the sense of the hospital team. Even when death seems to bring the task to an end, members of the primary health-care team may still deal with the aftermath of the trauma through other members of the family or neighbourhood.

In addition, we have seen that people's expectations regarding health and their attendant attitudes have also changed. When people become patients, these different attitudes can affect the expectations that they have of the professionals who take care of them when they are ill. In general the population is better educated, increasingly more health-conscious; less likely to be content with taking a passive role in relation to the treatment or management of their illnesses; less likely to be content to be silenced, baffled or impressed by the medical languages of mystification. They are also more likely to conceive of their illnesses as a result of a complex interaction of environmental, social, psychological and physical factors.

In order to deliver a health-care service the various professionals involved must be able to communicate and collaborate with each other. Shared goals and inter-professional respect and recognition are prerequisites for the successful delivery of health care. The very question of 'successful' health delivery has also been transformed. For we can no longer confine ourselves to concepts of 'cure'. Through the chronicity of incurable, degenerative diseases 'cure' has been transmuted to 'care' . . . the quality of the patients' lives whilst they are ill has become the focus of much of the team's work.

Differences of opinion within the team are usually experienced as personality conflicts. The truth is that inter-professional perception and inter-professional communication are as much affected by the general culture and the history and the status of the participating occupations as by the intrinsic personalities of those who wear the hat of doctor, nurse or social worker.

Different occupations: different views of the world

Man . . . has a vital interest in retaining his frame of orientation. His capacity to act depends upon it and in the last
analysis, his sense of identity. If others threaten him with ideas
that question his own frame of orientation, he will react to those
ideas as if to a vital threat.

Eric Froman, *The Anatomy of
Human Destructiveness*, (1972)

The contributing professions to health care each have a distinct
occupational culture. Not only are their contributing roles different, as are their pecuniary rewards and their social status; but so
are their styles of learning different. Bligh (1979) concludes that,
as a result, there is a stark contrast in their constructions of
reality.[23]

Each profession acts in a sense like a tribe. Members are
nurtured in distinctive ways, they develop their concepts in
exclusive gatherings (called professional training, or college membership), they have their own leaders and pecking orders. Like all
tribal societies they impose sanctions on non-conforming members. If a member takes on the reality constructs of another tribe,
then they may even be threatened with exclusion.

In her 1987 paper Huntingdon suggests that an occupational
culture is made up of its sense of mission, aim and task; the focus
and orientation of the profession; its ideological knowledge base
and its technology; its status and prestige; its orientation to clients
and patients and its orientation to other professions.[24] Certainly if
one compares these indicators between nurses and doctors, social
workers and nurses, or doctors and social workers, there are
distinct and potentially irreconcilable differences in their
occupational identity constructs.

My own research (1990) with undergraduate trainees in all
three professions indicates that there are already clear and distinct
occupational identities at a relatively early stage of professional
development.[25] More seriously, however, even at this early stage
there are strongly negative stereotyped perceptions of the other
professions. The sense of inclusion (we belong) and exclusion
(they don't); the gathering sense of 'Us' and 'Them' is basic to the
formation of a clear sense of group identity. What is worrying
about this research is the negative nature of the perceived differ-

ences. This augurs badly for the future when such trainees (with attitudes further hardened through exposure to their occupational culture and having been in receipt of the negative perceptions of other professions) are required to work together in a collaborative setting where issues of life and death are at stake.

Such stereotypic perception can only be ameliorated by exposure to and collaboration with the reality of the perceived 'out group'. Further research indicates that this should take place early in the training of health-care professionals. It should also continue throughout post-qualifying education and be framed in a way so that the unconscious tendency to stereotype can be made conscious, and thus consciously tested against reality.

It is highly unlikely that the educational changes required to make the shift from the 'expert' professional with his/her well-defined sense of autonomy and skills to the 'reflective' professional who is willing to share his/her authority and tolerate the uncertainty and frustration of team-work will be undertaken. Indeed the Griffiths Report on community care,[26] although allowing for a more flexible approach than is currently possible and calling for a full assessment of the training implications of the professionals involved, limits its recommendation on training to management skills.

The fundamental shift required in moving from an expert 'doctor-centred' health-care model to one where the focus is on the patient's needs as defined partly by the patient is a long way away. The patient may indeed be waking up and having a say but it would seem the ensuing 'conversation' resembles that of a shouting match rather than an orderly discussion where each side respects the skills, needs and status of the other.

7

The Planners Move In

Depending on your point of view, this chapter might have been included in the second section of this book as part of the solution as opposed to the problem. Certainly as far as the medical profession is concerned, the involvement of central government, bureaucratic agencies, health-care administrators, hospital managers and politicians of whatever hue in their affairs is seen as a problem. For many doctors this intrusion has not provided them with any solution with which they have felt comfortable. Whether or not the public has gained from the bureaucratisation of health care is difficult to gauge and the debate over the UK's present government's White Paper on the National Health Service and the effect of the internal market on patient satisfaction will not be known for several years. Its implementation in 1990, however, and the fierce and at times vitriolic exchanges between the Secretary of State for Health and the leaders of the medical profession were the nadir of the profession's relationship with any government. A Tory government appeared to have managed to produce the sort of control over the medical profession that the Socialist Medical Association had been campaigning for for years:

> A Labour Government will need to challenge (continually) the validity of professional activity from the State's cost-effectiveness viewpoint. Are the things the profession do worthwhile? Are particular clinical activities being neglected even though they would almost certainly be useful and effective, whilst less useful practices are continued. . . . To influence the application of health sciences in this way, we will need more than a strong DHSS that controls the distribution of resources. The local use of resources, the choice of options demand a local challenge to the alliance of professional and commercial interest from knowledgeable and articulate public bodies.[1]

How did the medical profession arrive at a situation where both Conservative and Labour political thinkers involved with health care came to the same conclusion – the medical profession's stranglehold on the practice of medicine had to be broken once and for all if effective planning was to be introduced. The World Health Organisation had gone one step further and advocated the de-professionalisation of primary care as the most important single step in raising national health levels.[2] To understand how this state of affairs has arisen one needs to trace the historical and fairly recent intrusion of central government in matters of health.

The bureaucratisation of medicine

Medical bureaucracy began with the emergence of the hospital. These institutions originated as part of the charitable and religious works of mediaeval monasteries. They were the original 'hospitiums' or guest houses for pilgrims travelling to holy shrines. These early institutions were open to all – the infirm, young, old and poor. Gradually they took on more specialised roles and the emergence of lunatic asylums, the leprosarium and the 'lying in' hospital became relatively common. A survey of 1719 revealed that twenty-three English counties had no hospitals, but by 1798 nearly every large town had established an infirmary with the aid of a private benefactor.[3] The nineteenth century saw two major developments: the further specialisation of hospitals and the beginning of government control. The passion for facts and knowledge, characteristic of this century, allowed for the emergence of the doctor as 'sociologist'. Armed with accurate figures, it was possible to demonstrate the effect of social class, unemployment, poverty and poor housing on health status. The beginning of the influence of central government on doctors and patients commenced. Until then the major legal and governmental decrees involved the education of doctors and the granting of licences. Now government, like the Church before it, became involved in controlling tasks that doctors could or would not perform. Legislation concerning the spread of infection, the Poor Law Reform, the control of public sewage, all became legitimate areas for central control and formed the basis for the development of the public health and hygiene movement.

Meanwhile the growth in both number and size of hospitals brought with it a need for a bureaucratic structure and central authority. However, hospitals were not a typical bureaucratic institution, for they possessed a dual system of authority. The administrative structure was managed separately from the professional task of caring for the patients, and doctors retained not only their administrative autonomy but were able to control the lay managers as well.

The Crimean War, the Boer War and the First World War brought about major changes in the medical provisions of the country, not least because the government discovered that the male population in Britain suffered from a number of disabling diseases which limited recruitment into the armed forces. In addition, the hospital facilities were unable to cope with the large-scale casualties of modern warfare. Nevertheless in 1917 it was safer to be a soldier in France than a baby in England: over 1,000 infants under the age of one year died every week in England.[4] Prepaid medical care had begun to be available to trade union members through the friendly societies or mutual benefit societies and other such institutions, but it was not until 1911 when the Liberal Prime Minister, Lloyd George, introduced the National Health Insurance Act that the beginnings of a National Health Service began. This Act allowed for the free treatment of all men and women in employment, and by 1948 the number of eligible people had risen to 25 million. The first Ministry of Health was created in 1919 and Lord Dawson, an eminent physician and public figure, produced a report which extended free treatment to groups other than those in employment. However, even as late as 1920, it was still possible for a woman to have to seek medical assistance from up to five different doctors, depending on her financial situation and disease. Even though a very large proportion of hospitals were under local government control from the beginning of the twentieth century, there was no systematic and general distribution of health provision throughout the country. Before the National Health Service in 1948, there were up to 400 different contributory schemes covering payment of hospital bills.

The Poor Law had been abolished in 1929 and, with the impetus of the Second World War and the developments in medical technology and treatment, the groundwork was laid for the *Beveridge Report* which advocated the founding of a National Health Service. The BMA, although advocating a comprehensive health service, resisted the Labour government throughout the passage of the Bill, and was able to ensure that medical autonomy was preserved. Aneurin Bevan's success in pushing through his reforms was partly as the result of his ability to drive a wedge between the consultants and the general practitioners. Consultants were offered hospital contracts which ensured they had managerial control, whilst at the same time they were allowed to continue in private practice. General practitioners were given the status of independent contractors, had 50 per cent representation on the Executive Committees (Family Practitioner Committees), which were their administrative bodies, and avoided a salaried service. Thus the National Health Service, although extending free treatment to everyone, both in the community and in hospitals, was largely fashioned and certainly administered in such a way that the medical profession retained both control and autonomy.

The Socialist belief that, by providing free and universal care, the demand for health care would gradually reduce as the population's standard of health improved, was soon recognised as totally unfounded. Indeed the opposite situation developed where increased demand meant that fixed budgeting for the Health Service was an impossible option. The Fifties were a difficult time for Britain generally, and the Health Service, although widely welcomed, suffered from lack of expansion and investment. The Conservatives returned to power in 1951 having won the political argument that the inflation of health care costs was far higher than that predicted by Labour. Although wanting to introduce reforms, the Conservatives recognised the popularity of the NHS and chose inactivity.

Meanwhile hospitals developed under a tripartite system of control, the matron in charge of the nurses, the medical superintendent organising medical care, and the lay administrator involving himself with the day-to-day running of the hospital. There was no doubt as to who was in charge, as the title 'medical superintendent' indicated, although this title was not always used. Similarly within the community, the medical officer of health was responsible for all welfare services provided by the local authorities. The Fifties were also a very difficult time for general practitioner services. The rigid remuneration system, the lack of any financial support for premises or ancillary staff meant that, by 1960, the number of general practitioners had actually diminished – list sizes had grown, and there was a great danger that this branch of the medical profession would disappear. The status and pay of consultants were at their highest, and to enter general practice meant that for most doctors they had 'fallen off the ladder'. The Charter for a Family Doctor Service in 1964 revolutionised the organisation and pay of general practitioners and marked the beginning of a renaissance in this discipline. The granting of a Royal Charter to the College of General Practitioners in 1967 further enhanced the standing of this branch of the profession. It was achieved also with little or no loss of independence.

The hospitals remained relatively well-staffed in the Fifties and a report on future medical staffing needs incorrectly advised a reduction in medical school places and paved the way for the understaffing crisis of the Sixties and Seventies. There developed an influx of immigrant doctors to fill the vacancies created partly by the inadequate supply of British graduates and partly because of the high level of emigration to Canada and the United States by doctors wishing to maintain both status and pay, which were beginning to be eroded. Nevertheless, the medical profession's hold on recruitment and the structure of medical schools was still unchallenged. The following quote from the evidence submitted by the Royal College of Surgeons to the Pilkington Committee (1958) about entry to medical training illustrates the culture fostered by many teaching hospital consultants.

> There has always been a nucleus in medical schools of students from cultured homes. This nucleus has been responsible for the continued high social prestige of the profession as a whole and for the maintenance of medicine as a learned profession. Medicine would lose immeasurably if the proportion of such students were to be reduced in favour of the precocious children who qualify for subsidies from Local Authorities and the State purely on examination results.[5]

Teaching hospital consultants, because of their prestige and power, ensured not only that the 'right sort' of student was accepted into medical school but that the numbers were reduced to ensure that the status of consultants remained intact.

The 1960s saw a major expansion in hospital building which continued into the Seventies. However, the rising costs of the Health Service had by now become an acute level of concern for all major political parties. A crucial consequence of this expansion was the development of the NHS as the biggest employer in Europe. Health care had become a labour intensive industry and the ancillary health worker through his union was demanding a say in the pay structure and thus helped to determine resource allocation. Again, through his union, the ancillary health worker, who previously had been under the control of the medical super-intendent, was able to remove himself from his direct authority and, from around the mid-Sixties, lay management and hospital administration began to develop its own discipline and career structure. When the Seebohm Report (1969) advocated the separation of social services from health, the figure of the lady almoner gradually disappeared and the social worker appeared on the health-care scene, fiercely protecting her independence.[6] Social work, as a discipline, was very heavily influenced by the radical ideas of the Sixties and took on what seemed to most doctors an overtly hostile approach to medicine. The medical officer of health was replaced by the community physician and yet another area of medical hegemony was seen to disappear. The Salmon Report (1966) on senior nursing staff structure introduced the concept of the manager-nurse and ensured that nurses who had been excluded from Hospital Management Committees would be given a more effective voice.

> Nurses appear to occupy a secondary position. This stems from the incoherence of the nursing administration itself and a seeming inability on the part of the nurses themselves to assert the rights of their emergent profession.[7]

Meanwhile the consultants who had not yet recognised the consequences of these changes accepted new responsibilities with regard to management structures within the hospitals. Each specialty would be organised within divisions and would under-take the review of resources (bed allocation, junior hospital posts) required for their particular specialty. Medical power was still very influential and in obstetrics the male obstetricians almost managed to eliminate the independence of the female midwifery service and ensured that it functioned under the control of the consultants.

The Seventies were the decade when the planners finally moved into the Health Service in force. Both Labour and Con-servative governments sought to control expenditure within the NHS and efficiency and cost-effectiveness became the guiding principles for the reorganised structure. A three-tiered structure of region, area and district administrative levels over which the DHSS assumed overall command was introduced. The number of committees grew exponentially and business methods and delegation downwards were introduced in an attempt to rationalise the decision-making process.

The medical profession nevertheless still retained the largest grouping of seats on the Regional Authorities, but for the first time there was an influx of commercial and business representation: Family Practitioner Committees still had a 50 per cent medical membership and the all-powerful committee that could help it control levels of expenditure and distribute them more equitably between the hospital and community health services and the Resource Allocation Working Party (RAWP) came into existence. At the same time the consumer was finally given an opportunity to have an official voice in the running of the Health Service and the Community Health Councils appeared on the scene. These lacked any effective power but their emergence allowed for the complaints procedures against doctors to be more effectively articulated and encouraged the appearance of the Parliamentary Commissioner, or Health Ombudsman, whose task was to examine complaints made against the administrative and non-clinical areas of the Health Service.

The Seventies were also the decade of union militancy, especially within the Health Service that had so far escaped the problems that had beset other nationalised industries. The low pay in a predominantly female work-force from Commonwealth countries had ensured a compliant work-force, often with the collusion of the trade unions themselves. However, the increased militancy that was present in other unions spread to the Health Service and the two major unions, COHSE (Confederation of Health Service Employees) and NUPE (National Union of Public Employees), began to co-operate first over nurses' pay and eventually over the pay of the ancillary workers. For the first time within the Health Service selective strikes occurred which ended in the infamous 'winter of discontent', and finally the demise of the Labour government.

The DHSS had taken to planning as a way of avoiding these crises and had commissioned a wide-ranging report which was to plan for NHS spending in cycles of 10–15 years. These strategic plans were published in *Priorities for Health and Personal Social*

Services in England in 1976, and for the first time the idea of fixed budgets and cash limits was introduced into the managerial thinking of the now ever-increasing army of hospital administrators. Several independent reports were concluding that all was not well with the British National Health Service. The *Black Report* (1980)[8] and the *Acheson Report* (1989)[9] identified major health discrepancies throughout the country which reflected social class, economic status and occupational groupings. Health-care delivery services within the inner cities were of a much lower standard than those found in other parts of the country and it was clear that not only was there a funding crisis, but there was also a health-care crisis within the Health Service. The medical profession, which had joined the militancy of the Health Service unions in the mid-Seventies, now found unity in blaming the government for its poor planning and inadequate funding. The work undertaken by RAWP was seen to be ineffective and wasteful, and ward and hospital closures were the clear evidence of the failure of central government. Unfortunately the profession had little to offer as an alternative other than the pious statement that the profession should be allowed to 'get on with the job'. This it was clear was not going to happen, and the election of the Thatcher government in 1979 was to produce a major rethink of the organisation of the Health Service, that is likely to prove the most radical since its inception.

The White Paper (1989)

Two of the seemingly inviolate aspects of the medical profession's relationship with successive governments were their clinical autonomy and financial independence. Doctors assumed and insisted that they, and they alone, could determine the standards of medical and surgical care which their patients received. Clinical freedom meant that they could choose to prescribe whatever drug they chose and perform whatever operation or procedure they felt appropriate. Patients were able to redress any 'mistakes' through the courts and doctors were subject to 'peer pressure' as to what was and what was not an acceptable clinical procedure. This loose and informal procedure was felt to work well and has been the accepted method of making doctors accountable. Any attempts to change or tamper with clinical autonomy have always been unsuccessful even when initiated by the profession.

The Royal College of General Practitioners in a document surprisingly similar to the government's discussion paper, *Primary Health Care* (1986), suggested the introduction of a 'Good Practice Allowance'. This was criticised harshly by members of the College and the authors described as elitist and 'out of touch'. When the government introduced its discussion document, the majority of the profession assumed it would be defeated as easily as the College's initiative had been. However, the government was intending not only to introduce some clinical control over the doctors' work but to make the whole service more 'financially accountable'. This latter intent received as much if not more criticism from the profession, and stimulated the Secretary of State for Health to make his controversial remark that he wished that doctors 'would not start feeling for their wallets' when he mentioned reform. It is interesting to place this remark alongside Bevan's when he introduced the NHS in 1948; he was heard to comment that he had to 'line the consultants' pockets with gold'. For although consultants were on salaried contracts which made them employees, the details of these contracts made it almost impossible to terminate them; they were able to continue in private practice and award themselves their own 'merit awards' which for some could often double their salaries. On the other hand, general practitioners were classified as self-employed even though nearly 100 per cent of their pay came from NHS sources. This 'self-employed' status has been very jealously guarded and has meant that the contractual agreement with the employing authority (Family Practitioner Committee) was almost non-existent and rarely enforceable. Roy Griffiths, when asked to review the doctors' contract for the government, was heard to say 'What contract?' However, it was not only the contractual base with doctors that the government wished to alter. The seemingly open-ended budget available to the NHS and ability of medicine to develop and demand more expensive machines leading to more opportunities for diagnosis, early treatment and replacement surgery meant that revenue planning and resource allocation were impossible tasks. In an attempt to address this problem, the government has introduced proposals in the White Paper to give hospitals an opportunity to become 'self-governing' and 'self-financing' and general practitioners an opportunity to maintain their own practice budgets.

The introduction of 'the internal market' into the National

Health Service is viewed by the government as an essential part of its ability to control costs and, it is thought, improve the services. As yet it is far too early to know whether this financial experiment will work or not. The BMA's immediate response was almost entirely critical and apart from acknowledging a need for 'medical audit', it began an intense and costly campaign in an attempt to defeat the government and prevent the introduction of the White Paper. Meeting after meeting indicated that the large majority of the profession was against the proposal. Even when, after prolonged negotiation, the BMA recommended acceptance of the new general practitioner contract, the voting membership (all GPs in the UK) rejected the advice of its representatives by a majority of two to one. Mass resignations were threatened and it appeared that the doctors had the support of their patients, the nursing profession, the Community Health Councils and the Royal Colleges, as well as the opposition parties. The government, however, won its case where it mattered – in Parliament – the National Health Service and Community Care Bill is to be introduced in 1990. Putting aside the political and economic arguments, it appears that the medical profession has, for the first time, to come under a system of accountability, both clinical and financial, that has never been present in its history.

Under the new contract, general practitioners will be expected to provide services to their patients about which in the past they alone determined the necessity, e.g., GPs will be required to offer a medical check to all new registrations within six weeks of registering, and the details of what the check-up should include are laid down in their contract. Since their inception, Family Practitioner Committees (now called Family Health Service Authorities) have acted as an administrative office with few if any managerial or supervisory powers. Under the new arrangements they will be in a position to monitor and determine the prescribing patterns of a doctor as well as his willingness to undertake immunisation and other preventive measures. Even more critical for the doctors is that the management structures of these new Family Health Service Authorities will no longer have a 50 per cent medical membership, so that ultimate control has been well and truly removed from the doctors. The hospital situation is less clear but the dual managerial structure referred to earlier in the chapter has already been eroded and consultants have found it increasingly difficult to be in sole control of their waiting lists, operating times and budget allocation. One of the assumptions underpinning the government's plans is that the increasing financial accountability at a local hospital level will enable 'inefficient consultants' to be identified and, if required, disciplined. If the Labour Party wins the 1992 election, it will be very interesting to observe how many of the changes now being introduced would actually be repealed. The Labour Party has always wanted to erode the monopoly of power over the nation's health that doctors have so far possessed. They may well choose to repeal some of the 'internal market' aspects of the new law but are likely to accept with glee the fact that the medical profession has so clearly lost the battle with the government and consequently surrendered much of its power. The effect of these changes has left many doctors, both old and young, demoralised and uncertain. Resignations from the Health Service are increasing and not necessarily for financial reasons. The need to be in control and in charge has at times a greater hold on doctors than financial security, especially when that security is dependent on meeting targets and reporting to lay managers.

Most of these changes have been proposed with the assumption that the patient will benefit. Indeed both the medical profession's and the government's arguments had the patient either worse off or much better off.

The government's White Paper was labelled *Working for Patients* and the BMA's advertising campaign highlighted how patients would suffer through having to travel, to obtain the 'best buy', or through not being able to obtain a drug because their GP had expended all his allocated budget. These tactics are part of the negotiating game, but, in this case, the football is the patient and the consequences of the proposed changes are uncertain. It is salutary to note that Sir Kenneth Stowe, the Permanent Secretary at the Department of Health, wrote after retiring in 1987: 'The White Paper is not an appraisal of 40 years of caring for the national health: the betterment in the health of the population at large is barely touched on, in nineteen words in the first paragraph.'[10] Earlier on he states: 'The ends of good health care and how best to attain them tend to be squeezed out because Ministers and their most senior officials are pre-occupied with central Government responsibility for the health authorities.'

What would Sir Kenneth have liked to have addressed more thoroughly in his time as Permanent Secretary, a time when the

Department was undertaking its most critical review of the NHS? Again he provides a list which suggests that the 'greening process' might have been accelerated had he been able to have more impact on the White Paper than it appears he had. The list Sir Kenneth provides include:

- Education for good health and self-help
- Medicines and self-medication
- The respective roles of the different clinical professions
- Medical education – the role of the universities, and of the teaching hospitals
- Research and development
- The caring community and its renewal
- An aged and ageing population
- The voluntary sector
- Representing the patient's interests.

Very few if any of these items have been directly addressed by the White Paper, for it is clear that the changes about to be introduced have more to do with altering the power relationship between central government and the medical profession than 'the betterment in the health of the population at large'. The consequences of this shift in the power-relationship may well be to the patient's benefit but it has left both individual doctors and the medical profession disillusioned and demoralised.

8

The Profession Reacts

In 1975, the Merrison Committee of Inquiry into the Regulation of the Medical Profession wrote: 'Nobody who has seen the detailed evidence presented to us would underestimate the nature and scale of the problems of the sick doctor.'[1] Fourteen years later, a junior hospital doctor went to the High Court because he felt that he was having to work unreasonable hours and that his working conditions were unhealthy. These two events illustrate the scale of the problem, for it has been well known for several decades that there is an undue morbidity and mortality within the medical profession, yet the profession in almost a lemming-like response has failed to address the toll on its individual members. At the same time the profession as a whole and medicine as a discipline have been the subject of a number of serious and well-reasoned critiques which have not been answered adequately and which have left many new entrants into the profession unhappy and disillusioned well before their working careers have begun. Porter quotes the story of the young doctor who entered general practice and who then returned to his medical school to demand his money back as he had been so inadequately prepared for the job.[2] It is a well-accepted axiom that the period of vocational training for general practice is often an 'unlearning period' where newly trained doctors have to unlearn what they were taught at medical schools in order to allow them to work effectively within general practice.

The New York psycho-analyst who first used the term 'burn-out' was describing the emotional and physical exhaustion he witnessed amongst many of his medical patients.[3] It is now apparent that as a term it can be applied to several professional groups – nurses, social workers, teachers. The stages of burn-out include a period of initial enthusiasm followed by stagnation, frustration and apathy, and at different points in this downward spiral the casualties will present with a differing set of symptoms, partly dependent on the ethos and training that each profession has been given.

The morbidity figures that can be obtained for the medical profession illustrate the final chapter in some of their lives. Doctors have twice as many deaths from road accidents as the general population. In the US it is estimated that in 1976 there were between 13,600 and 22,000 alcoholics amongst the 324,000 doctors.[4] It is not possible to translate these figures to the British scene, but using figures from Scotland and death-rates from cirrhosis as a guide, the incidence of alcoholism amongst doctors is about three times the expected figure for professional groups. The level of alcoholism only illustrates part of the problem. Alcohol has for a long time been a method of coping with stress amongst medical students and, out of a group of forty-one doctors treated for alcoholism, five had started drinking heavily at medical school.[5] As quoted by a doctor who became an alcoholic 'The more common daily ritual included an internment and carefully titrated feed of alcohol coupled with many mints or cough sweets. Some work suffered, particularly record-keeping and letter-writing.'

Mental illness, including depression and suicide, are twice as common amongst doctors as amongst men of equal professional standing, but accurate statistics are difficult to arrive at and it is clear that doctors intent on suicide are more able to obtain the means whereby to kill themselves than other groups.[6] Again, the stark figures for depression and suicide reveal only a small section of the problem: for many doctors, the issues are more to do with chronic fatigue, low-level distress, unhappiness, marital discord, divorce and disillusionment.

The typical junior hospital doctor in the UK is still working, on average, over 80 hours a week and for some 8 per cent this figure is 130 hours. Junior doctors have had to be on continuous duty for up to 56 hours and several have recorded that on occasions they have had less than two hours' unbroken sleep. The situation is allowed to continue in part because the senior members of the profession believe this to be a sort of 'rite of passage'. 'We did it when we were your age and look how successful we are now.' The recorded level of diagnostic errors, incorrect prescribing and more serious surgical mistakes is difficult to ascertain for obvious reasons, but anecdotal evidence and the personal experience of many doctors suggest that if the facts concerning the level of inefficiency and dangerous practice were to become more widely known, then the public would demand some urgent changes. In part, because the medical profession and individual doctors continue to uphold the view that like the Pope the infallibility of the doctor, once lost, would undermine the whole 'faith', the situation continues. However the pressure for change is now coming from within the medical profession itself and the group cohesion is no longer so apparent as it was. In previous decades many doctors delayed getting married until they had obtained a consultant's post or a practice. With increasingly fewer doctors willing to follow this pattern, many medical marriages that begin during the early years of training fail and end in divorce. The long hours, the frequent change in jobs and hospitals, the need to respond to emergencies and the constant interruption of the telephone, can play havoc with the needs of a young couple embarking on married life. In 1983 Gerber conducted a study of medical marriages and two quotes help to illustrate the problems from both the male-husband-doctor's perspective as well as from the female-wife-home-maker:[7]

> I'm so tired all the time. I can't even be by myself, let alone with anyone else. At first, going home to Nancy was like heaven, a refuge from all this. But it's hard to go home, get used to that and re-enter this world at the hospital. You have to keep readjusting and you get to the point where you just don't want to or can't any more. It's easier just to be here so you're not torn by things at home. It's easier to be with the nurses, they know what it's like. There don't have to be any attachments. You don't have to give in the same way. Easier just not to think of home.

> I'm always conscious that if I criticise my husband's compulsive dedication to work I will be regarded as a spoiled princess. When I have to attend a family gathering or a friend's cocktail party by myself – which is quite often – people will just ooh and aah after they learn my husband's absence is due to the fact that he had to deliver a baby – 'How terrific', they'll say, 'You must be so proud'. I'm in the position of having to smile appreciatively about his accomplishments when deep down I'm really resenting the closeness between my husband and that other woman giving birth.

In a more recent survey an understanding of how the health of a spouse is affected by the husband's compulsive work-load was apparent in one respondent:

> I wonder how often ill health presenting in the spouse is a reflection of the state of mind of their partner. I sought help when my own wife became seriously depressed and was unable to care for our children. In the course of therapy, it became clear that I was the one generating a great deal of the domestic stress and disharmony. The problems are the difficulties of combining a demanding job which often intrudes into a normal family life.[8]

The increasing awareness of this intrusion on normal family life has been heightened in recent years as more and more women enter medical school and have to face the triple problem of being a doctor, a wife and a mother. Over 50 per cent of a group of 111 women doctors studied in America showed signs of significant psychological disorder and 33 per cent were depressed.[9] The problem for women medical students is particularly acute as they lack the role models – there are very few women consultants in teaching hospitals, and thus have to adapt and conform to the stereotype of the male medical student.

At the same time as the doctors begin to acknowledge their own struggle to maintain their powerful persona, other health care professionals are demanding a degree of autonomy and independence that ensures that the unquestioned authority of the doctor will no longer go unchallenged. The nursing profession has sought hard to relinquish the Nightingale tradition of the 'handmaiden' to the doctor. Nursing as a profession has subordinated itself to the medical profession, so that nurses were trained to 'carry out the doctor's orders'. With the increase in specialisation in both medicine and nursing, it became clear that nurses were far more able than newly qualified doctors in performing certain skilled tasks. Even with the confidence of both superior knowledge and unique skills, nurses have found it difficult to obtain a degree of professional autonomy. In the last five years, however, the concept of the nurse-practitioner seeing patients directly and being able to prescribe has been proposed.[10] Recent surveys suggest that nurses are no longer willing to follow medical instructions unquestioningly.[11] It is clear that the stereotyping between nurses and doctors occurs even before they graduate. Joint seminars between medical and nursing students reveal a level of distrust and hostility which explains all too graphically why, once qualified, health-teams do not work well. The medical profession and individual doctors are viewed by student nurses as being autocratic, authoritarian, macho, busy, not willing to listen and generally unsympathetic towards patients. Whereas nurses would would be reluctant to voice these complaints openly, it is increasingly the case that the nursing profession has adopted a more overtly critical and feminist attitude towards the medical profession. The not dissimilar situation has occurred amongst social workers, clinical psychologists, community psychiatric nurses, pharmacists and, more recently, alternative and complementary practitioners. The inability, and at times unwillingness, of the medical profession to meet the needs of the patient has meant that the other professions engaged in health care have come forward to fill the gap.

> Pharmacists eager to extend their activities in hospital in a clinical direction have moved into those areas where medical practitioners have previously tended to take short cuts or have neglected entirely. For example patient counselling, monitoring of drug side-effects and the provision of drug information services.[12]

The British Medical Association's survey on alternative medicine identified, amongst other factors, the fact that patients sought help from such practitioners because of the amount of time they were given and the willingness to listen.[13] Both these factors are the first casualties in the life of a busy, overworked and stressed doctor. Voting with their feet, patients are finding health-care practitioners who will offer them what they consider to be essential ingredients of a good doctor–patient relationship – warmth, empathy and a willingness to listen.

Further blows to the prestige of doctors and medicine as a discipline have come from sociologists, anthropologists, philosophers, scientists and eminent critics from within the profession itself. Some of these have been referred to earlier but a more detailed description of these criticisms will illustrate how deeply troubled medicine has become as an academic, let alone scientific, discipline.

Ivan Illich, an agent-provocateur of many professions, rocked the medical world in 1976 with his book *Medical Nemesis* which was later entitled *Limits to Medicine*.[14] His first title drew on the Greek myth of Prometheus who stole fire from the heavens and through his greed, presumption and arrogance (hubris) brought about his own downfall – his nemesis. Illich's principal statement was that 'the medical establishment had become a major threat to health'. Its 'hubris' at assuming it could heal and cure all man's ills had inevitably brought its repercussions and that its nemesis and downfall were overdue. He amassed an impressive array of supportive research to show how much of modern medical treatment was not only useless but harmful. Amongst the many indictments were that 15 per cent of all hospital admissions are the result of a medically-induced disease, 7 per cent of all hospital admissions result in some compensatable injury. As I have mentioned, he labelled this aspect of the epidemic of modern medicine clinical iatrogenesis. He then went on to illustrate how the medical profession influences the health policies of various countries and has a disproportionate control on how money is spent on health care and, more importantly, where it is spent. He pointed out that because doctors in hospitals are interested in high technology medicine, a disproportionate part of health budgets is spent on medical equipment to the detriment of preventive and community services. He saw the development of coronary care units and the purchase of high-cost machines, 'scans' and linear accelerators as the direct result of the medical profession's interest rather than because they necessarily benefited the consumer. He quoted de Kadt's *Inequality and Health*: 'Professional ideologies that focus on the maintenance of high standards of medical care keep in being a health system which neglects the simple needs of the many in order to concentrate on the complex and costly conditions of a few.'[15]

The consequence of this has been explored more fully earlier.

In *The Role of Medicine* (1979), Thomas McKeown chose to adopt a more academic and less strident tone.[16] He avoided the 'doctor-bashing' remarks of *Limits to Medicine* and distanced himself from Illich. In his foreword, he writes: 'The two books [his and Illich's] have little in common except perhaps in the sense that the Bible and the Koran could be said to be identified by the fact that both are concerned with religious matters.' It is an interesting parallel and one which is quite telling. For like the Bible and the Koran, both books search for 'the truth' and what they uncover is not in any way dissimilar. McKeown's approach is to illustrate how, for most diseases, prevention by control of their origins is cheaper, more humane and more effective than intervention by treatment after they occur. McKeown viewed medical practice through a cultural and sociological framework and, like many observers before him and subsequent to him (*Black Report*, 1982), found that class divisions, poverty, poor education, inadequate housing, unemployment, were all far more important factors in the causation of disease than viruses, bacteria and twisted molecules. The medical profession, both in its approach to understanding disease and treating it, failed to recognise the poverty and limitation of the bio-medical model which excluded psychology and social factors.

Ian Kennedy, in his book *The Unmasking of Medicine* (1981) which followed his Reith Lecture, describes some of the myths and fallacies that surround the way in which medical decisions, both clinical and political, are made. He examined the relationship between doctor and patient from an ethical, legal and philosophical perspective.[17] As a result of his own writings, the new 'specialty' of medical ethics developed. Kennedy drew attention to the political nature of the decisions surrounding the purchase of a kidney machine, the building of an old people's home and the ever-increasing drug bill.

These three books, amongst several others, confronted the medical profession with a view of itself it at once denied but at the same time recognised. The profession could no longer remain aloof and separate from such debates. However it has been unable to respond and adapt – undergraduate medical education has remained almost unchanged for decades and medical students are not being given the opportunity to integrate these criticisms of their discipline into their education.

The basic assumptions that underlie any system of medical care and medical education arise out of the cultural/philosophical and scientific beliefs that predominate in that society. As basic shifts occur in these assumptions, there needs to be a review of the current educational training offered, be it in medicine, physics or business. There have been many articles, numerous reports, several books, all drawing attention to the alleged deficiencies in current medical education. Some of these criticisms go back such a long way that it is pertinent to ask whether change can take place at all. In 1844 a working party of the BMA noted that 'no inconsiderable number of recently qualified men have no idea of the real duties of general practitioners until they are actually engaged in practice; many of them discover that their work is hardly that which they had anticipated'. Many of the difficulties encountered by doctors on first entering general practice have to do with the very specialised nature of the problems they see at teaching hospitals. Every month, of 1,000 adults, 750 will develop a symptom of some kind. Of those 750, 250 will go to their general practitioner, and 10–15 will be referred to hospital and 1–2 will be seen at a teaching hospital.[18] The patients and morbidity patterns that students see is therefore skewed awkwardly, and it can be hard for them to adjust to the realities of clinical presentation and 'abnormal' medical pathology, when they have to enter practice in other settings. Several authors have written on the socialisation process of medical school. Attention has been drawn to the loss of idealism that occurs and how the pre-clinical and clinical years can often become the pre-cynical and cynical years.[19] Medical training has a profound effect on social attitudes and some authors suggest that the selection of medical students is biased towards academic distinction and that the latter is a poor indicator of a good doctor.

In a study comparing attitudes of new medical students with students in arts and sciences, the medical students scored significantly lower than the other students on their ability to tolerate change, uncertainty and lack of structure.[20] A constellation of certain personality attributes seems to be more common amongst medical students, which may suggest that selection does indeed favour a particular set – or, as has been suggested, that selectors 'choose in their own image' so that the process repeats itself. This may indeed be true as very few non-specialists are involved in selection and the lay representation is almost absent. The characteristics identified as being present amongst both doctors and medical students include a preference for conventional values and willingness to accept uncritically the views of 'the authority'. There is too a lack of empathy with minority groups – blacks, homosexuals and, ironically, patients. There is a general 'tough-mindedness' towards such things as pain, drug-abuse and evidence of human weakness, and in contrast a lack of sensitivity and general rejection of emotions of tenderness or vulnerability. It would seem that medical students, if not 'tough' by the time they get to medical school, will have to 'toughen up' in order to become doctors. Yet it is clear that they are not all like that and that, for many, the years of their training are not only a disappointment but a major failure in education. A sample of statements made by students in the last five years illustrates the depth and tragedy of the failure of their teachers:

We are often dragged around the wards behind doctors and nurses who don't really like us being there. We stand around the bed and are taught on patients, and our embarrassment at times on behalf of what the person may be going through surrounded by our multitude, often prevents us from learning what is being taught. We also often have to go back afterwards to try and tell the patient what all the discussion was about because he is left in the air not really knowing.

I originally thought it was just a question of personality but now I see that sometimes considerateness, kindness and understanding, which really should be the basis of it all, are bred out of one.

Consultants do centre on physical signs and symptoms with aims of symptom relief. Virtually no encouragement is given re. life-style and education for living.

There is this contrast between goals and objectives that we are given at the beginning and what we actually see happening on the ward. We are told that we need to take into account what may happen to a patient when he goes home, but week after week, we see the emphasis on drug prescriptions and it is the lucky ones who have attention paid to the care they will receive on leaving hospital. A lot of our education is a waste of time and our enthusiasm. The methods we are assessed by are not relevant to health caring.

Everything is so hierarchical – there is no remnant of the apprenticeship for learning. We keep meeting the obstacle of entrenched tradition and closed minds. There is no outlet for the shock that many of us feel when meeting some of the diseases and hopelessness that is inevitable in the field of medicine specifically when meeting death. There is such a range of response from the pious to the ridiculous, and it is so difficult to accept the different responses of people who don't respond my way. There seems no means of dealing with this – it is so isolating.

They laugh at us when we even mention the possibility that an alternative form of medicine may help. We are taught all this technology. That's all very well, sometimes useful, but sometimes I feel if you take this away I won't be left with half a skill to deal with a patient.[21]

It is a sad reflection on the future of medicine in this country that little if any change has occurred even with these clear and poignant remarks. Attempts by distinguished academics (retired) to influence change have also proved futile. An open letter to the GMC by such a group in 1984 summarised the current criticisms levelled at medical education and referred to the GMC recommendation on the undergraduate curriculum in 1957. They drew attention to the way in which these recommendations have been largely ignored and highlighted two basic deficiencies:[22]

We believe that British medical education is failing in two respects:– firstly, in the extent to which it equips doctors with the capacity to think critically for themselves; and secondly in the degree to which it inculcates a broad holistic and sensitive outlook towards the health of both individuals and communities.

The letter goes on to elaborate on these two deficiences and describes the many factors that have prevented medical education from changing. These factors include:

(a) the lack of resources, both buildings and staff;
(b) appointment of academic staff pays little attention to knowledge and experience of education in comparison to research and clinical experience;
(c) the attitude of medical teachers is mostly to instruct and not to educate;
(d) the attitude of medical students suggests they prefer the dogmatic teaching styles which avoid the need for reflection, ambiguity and uncertainty;
(e) departmental teaching, often unco-ordinated, produces splintered learning, especially if no clear educational objectives exist;
(f) the pressure of work has required students to become observers of medical care, rather than participators, and that lack of direct patient experience leads to lack of proper integration of facts learned.

Although the authors of this letter suggest ways in which medical education can be improved, these are couched in terms that leave the basic structure of the five-year undergraduate curriculum intact. As medical students struggle with the enormous amount of information required to pass exams, they begin to have some of their idealism blunted by the many hours of hard work required. When they eventually go on the wards, they meet patients who are ill, but also who are anxious, frightened, depressed, angry and at times, rude and difficult. They see patients in pain, in tears and witness the last breath of a human being as he struggles for his life.

The instruction and guidance they get is not on how to handle these difficult human situations. Rather, they are asked about the state of the patient's liver or the latest blood test. They are expected to know when the last article on some new investigation was written. There is no doubt that this sort of instruction is essential – the high technical competence of our doctors is proof enough of that – but at what cost?

As the students struggle, not only with having to amass a new set of knowledge, they are overwhelmed with feelings they do not understand. Even worse, they may stop feeling altogether as a protection from these difficulties.

Oliver Cape said 'the practice of medicine reflects the education of yesterday'. If we are to provide our students with the education they deserve, then we need to complement our medical education with activities that will allow them an opportunity to explore and understand these aspects of our work.

Such activities should include a comprehensive interviewing course; small group discussions and seminars on human sexuality, death and dying, human awareness and the value of healing. As yet there has been little serious debate as to the needs for future training, partly because there is still a firm belief that there is little wrong with the product produced by medical schools.

As we have seen in earlier chapters, the ability to think in 'wholes' and to relate to one's peers and colleagues as well as the environment, the development of one's own imaginative centre and the cultivation of an inner self with a lively sense of the mystery of life and the ability to tolerate uncertainty are some of the 'Green' characteristics. Medical education, with its emphasis on 'parts' and on the need for distinct entities in disease labelling, sees its causative base as increasingly molecular, and emphasises the importance of numeracy, measurement and the technological apparatus for arriving at precision; thus it is almost at the opposite pole of the Green movement. The consumer-patient is requiring a different approach from his doctor. Medical schools are the factory floor for future doctors: they are still producing the old model for which there is increasing evidence of a poor market uptake. If medical educators fail to change the assembly-line, then it will either be changed by others or increasing support for the development of another model of health-care worker – nurse/practitioner, alternative primary health practitioner will grow, and the 'old model doctor' will increasingly be bypassed by patients, other health-care workers and governments alike.

PART III

Attempts at Solutions

9

The Feminine Principle

In 1830 a group of American male medical students met to protest at the attempt by Harriat Hunt to attend lectures at Harvard Medical School. Their resolutions included 'Resolved that no women of true delicacy would be willing in the presence of men to listen to discussion of subjects that necessarily come under consideration of the students of medicine. Resolve that we object to having the company of any female forced upon us who is disposed to unsex herself and to sacrifice her modesty by appearing with men in the lecture room.'[1]

Since then there has been a gradual but steady increase in the number of women entering medicine. Quotas regulating places for women were abolished in 1970 and, by 1985, 45 per cent of all entrants to medical school were women. Nevertheless, men still predominate in those specialties that have high status and high income. Whilst the numbers of women doctors may be an important development in the influence of women in health-care, it is from the cultural and psychological shifts in attitudes that one can observe even more important changes.

Notwithstanding the presence of white witches, midwives and nurses, healing and health care have always been a male-dominated preserve. In Ancient Greece it was Apollo, the Sun God, and his son, Aesculapius, who became identified as the 'fathers' of medicine. Aesculapius was snatched from his mother's womb by Apollo and given to Chiron to bring up. From Chiron Aesculapius learnt his art and skill and became famous during the Trojan war, as did his two sons Podaliros (father of internal medicine) and Machaon (father of surgery). Aesculapius had a large family and his two daughters, Hygeia and Panacea, became associated with hygiene and treatment respectively. The development of the Aesculapian temples in Thessaly gradually spread throughout Greece and Rome, and, together with the influence of Hippocrates, formed the foundations of Western medicine.

The links between the Sun God Apollo, the Centaur Chiron, the Trojan warrior Aesculapius and medicine all help to empha- sise the aggressive nature of this branch of human endeavour. The language that is used, 'fighting disease', the 'battle against cancer', 'the magic bullet', 'stamping out infection' 'cutting out the growth', underpins the view that women are somehow inherently unsuited to the practice of medicine. Aesculapius was slain by Zeus for deigning to raise a man from the dead, thus challenging the Gods. Hades had complained to Zeus that his kingdom was being deprived of incumbents by Aesculapius' healing art and Zeus sent down a thunderbolt to slay the impudent mortal. The agony of Aesculapius' cries reached Zeus' ears and, with the consent of the other Gods, Aesculapius was raised from the dead to join the immortal Gods himself. The nature of Aesculapius' birth and death with the vivid description of transitions 'snatched from his dying mother's womb', 'raised from human physician to immortal God' illustrate graphically how the healers worked and lived on the boundaries of life and death.[2]

The symbolic representation of medicine and its link to mytho- logical themes is a crucial factor in the development and language that pervades medicine. Aesculapius' symbol of office, the serpent entwined around a staff, has emphasised the masculine nature of his craft. For, although the cosmology and symbolic significance of the serpent is large, it has primarily become associated with phallic power. The serpent is universally linked to pregnancy but, follow- ing the Jewish myth of the Garden of Eden, its link with trans- formation and rebirth is not so strong within Western cultures as is found in the East. The Aesculapian staff has one snake wound around a staff whilst the 'Caduceus', the symbolic representation found in India, Mesopotamia, Greece and Rome, has two snakes. In its full representation the Caduceus was a wand or staff surmounted by two wings or winged helmet. The wings symbolise transcendence, the wand is power, and the serpents represent healing and poison, illness and health. These are the com- plementary forces in nature – the union of both sexes. The Caduceus is the symbol of Mercury and Hermes, and its meaning is not so much related to its individual elements but to the composite nature of the whole. The Aesculapean staff and solitary snake does not possess the totality of meaning associated with the

Caduceus and is linked far more with power and energy than with transformation and complementarity.[3]

Thus the mythical symbols and language used to describe both anatomical and physiological processes have helped to shape medical approaches to women in health and in illness. The following examples illustrate how medicine inevitably partakes of the overall culture and society in which it operates.

Up until the late eighteenth century it was assumed that male and female bodies were structurally similar. The Bishop of Emesa

Figure 7 This nineteenth-century South Indian sculpture shows a minor female deity with the serpent of creative energy issuing from her vulva.

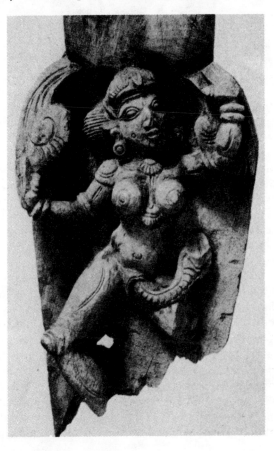

Figure 8 Georg Bartisch's illustration of phallus-like female reproductive organs (1575)

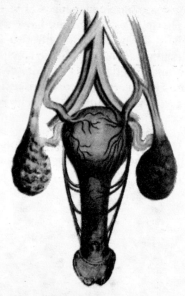

in Svria wrote in the fourth century: 'Women have the same genitalia as men except that theirs are inside the body and not outside it'.[4] As it became clear that this was not so, the difference between men and women was expressed in words and phrases that were male-dominated and ensured that the reader had no doubt as to which description was preferred.

Medical descriptions of menstruation, the menopause and reproductive processes all used language which helped to colour our attitudes in a particular direction. Havelock Ellis could write of women as being 'periodically wounded'.[5] Walter Heape, the Cambridge zoologist, in his description of menstruation used words like 'ragged wreck', 'torn glands', 'ruptured vessels', all conveying a traumatic event which as he puts it . . . 'would seem hardly possible to heal satisfactorily without the aid of surgical treatment'.[6] It is therefore not surprising that it used to be taught that 'menstruation is the uterus crying for a baby'.[7]

Menopause is described as a 'process of failure', the 'ovaries are shrunken', 'breasts and genitals atrophy', and it is not too difficult to comprehend why there is a widely accepted view that the menopause is a pathological process.[8] It is in highlighting the words and phrases found in medical text-books both past and present that the male bias towards women can be identified. This bias ensured that women's role in medicine was limited to that of the *comforting healer*. Female practitioners were few and far between and almost always attracted the opprobrium and disapproval of their male colleagues. Evidence of women as physicians is found in most cultures. They were often the wives or daughters of lower-order wound surgeons. In the fourteenth century, when the practice of medicine required licensure by examination, there were fifteen licensed female practitioners in Germany. It is only within obstetrics and the practice of midwifery that the woman practitioner was initially accepted by the male doctor. Before 1900 the majority of women were attended by other women during childbirth, although attitudes towards midwives were often expressed in the most extreme terms. Rosslin (1513), the first male author of a midwives' manual, wrote:

> I'm talking about the midwives all
> Whose births are empty as a hall
> And through their dreadful negligence
> Cause babies deaths devoid of sense
> So thus we see far and about
> Official murder there is no doubt.[9]

Figure 9 An illustration accompanying the late nineteenth-century biologist's account of what he saw as radical physiological distinctions between males and females, the male dominated by active, energetic katabolic functions and the female by passive, conservative anabolic functions (Geddes 1890)

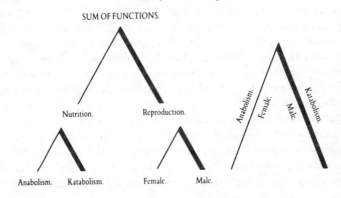

Figure 10 The symbol of the Caduceus (1515)

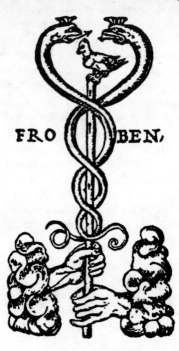

FRO   BEN,

Other views were more generous – 'As much as possible midwives managed deliveries by letting nature do the work.'[10] During the fifteenth and sixteenth centuries thousands of midwives were burnt at the stake as witches. The authoritative volume *Malleus Maleficarum* (The Hammer of Witches), written by two Franciscan monks detailed procedures as to how such midwives could be identified and persecuted. The midwives were associated with devil worship, and their craft, which involved the use of placentas, amniotic fluid and umbilical cords, began to disappear in the seventeenth century. In France, nationwide regulation of midwives was in place by 1726[11] and by 1800 most of central Europe was supplied with trained and qualified midwives. By this time, however, male doctors had begun to replace the midwife as the expert in matters dealing with pregnancy and birth and this trend continues to this day, although the medicalisation and male domination of women's bodies through health and illness has been challenged increasingly in the last two decades. The developments of modern care of the birthing process began with the realisation that infant mortality and maternal mortality rates were far too high. In 1870 maternal mortality figures suggested that one woman in every 120 died within four weeks of childbirth and the infant mortality was 150 per 1,000. Gradually the number of deliveries undertaken in hospital increased, so that the percentage of home births declined from 33 per cent in 1961 to only 3 per cent in 1976. Accompanying this development there arose an impressive array of procedures and interventions which emphasised the medical and surgical aspect of giving birth to the detriment of the human and personal. The inappropriateness and ineffectiveness of many of these procedures, including induction, foetal monitoring, shaving the vulva, the use of enemas, the wholesale use of anaesthesia and analgesics, the routine use of episiotomies and finally the rising incidence of Caesarian section, all involved giving more power to the obstetrician and less freedom to the woman, so that an obstetrician could write:

> Pregnancy is a state induced by the growth of a neoplasm; labour is a process accompanied by self-inflicted wounds and the puerperium is the period of healing – Midwifery concerns itself with the treatment of these three and is a pure surgical art. [12]

The premise that lay behind this medicalisation of perinatal care was that it resulted in a lowering of maternal mortality and increased the survival rate of new-born infants. Certainly the major improvement suggested in these figures coincided with what was seen as the capturing of the womb by the medical profession. It was not always clear whether these dramatic improvements were the result of social and educational changes together with the better housing and improved nutrition that occurred in the early part of this century. By the 1960s, however, the impersonal and technological model of perinatal care was being challenged by a number of individuals and consumer organisations. However, it was not only women who were challenging this medical domination. The standard of antenatal care as well as the birth process itself came in for criticism.

Morris, in a well-publicised paper, although agreeing with the need for safety and the hospitalisation of the pregnant woman, suggested that success should not always be measured in terms of

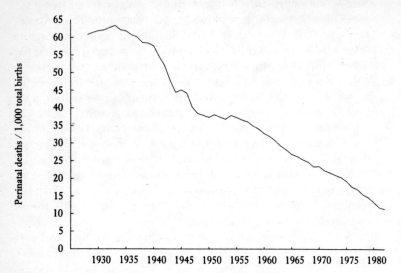

Figure 11 Perinatal mortality rates, England and Wales, 1928–82

Source: OPCS Mortality statistics, Series DH3 (Quoted in Ann Oakley, *The Captured Womb*)

life and death. He described the experience of antenatal clinics in a way that immediately struck a chord with many women.

> Women attend these clinics regularly, often as many as fourteen times. The clinic is usually drab and colourless, painted in bottle green, brown, or dirty cream. There are rows of uncomfortable benches. There is an atmosphere of coldness, unfriendliness, and severity more in keeping with the spirit of an income-tax office. The clinic is often overcrowded, and at best a crude appointment system is in operation. Despite this, women often wait 1–3 hours. The interview itself is usually extremely brief, and under such conditions there is little encouragement for the patient to ask questions or relieve herself of any nagging fears or doubts. Therefore she often remains in gross ignorance of what is happening to her. The doctors and nurses also remain virtual strangers since she rarely sees the same one at each visit.[13]

At the same time, women on both sides of the Atlantic were complaining, campaigning and writing about their experience of childbirth. Arms, in her book *Immaculate Deception* (1975), wrote 'I came out of the delivery numb from the waist to the

knees, dry and sour in the mouth, flat on my back and strapped to
a metal table four feet off the ground.'[14] Kitzinger, in her own
book *The Experience of Childbirth*,[15] reaffirmed many of these
descriptions and helped to strengthen the growing consumer
revolt which in Britain had begun with the National Childbirth
Trust in 1956. Advocates of natural childbirth espoused a model of
care that involved more human and personal contact during
antenatal care, a better informed and involved mother, a process
of delivery that was achieved without drugs, without interventions and where the mother retains control over herself and the
baby. AIMS (Association for Improvement in Maternity Services,
founded in 1960) and the Society for the Prevention of Cruelty to
Pregnant Women campaigned for freedom of choice and focused
less on the need for 'natural' childbirth.[16] The return of the midwife as a major figure in perinatal care was espoused as well as the
development of GP and community antenatal care. Gradually
the psychosocial aspects of care were acknowledged and fathers
were admitted to the delivery room. Routine practices such as
enemas and pubic shaving ceased. Pain control included the use of
breathing and relaxation skills learnt during antenatal clinics, and
there developed an understanding of the possible flexibility in

Figure 12 Maternal mortality rates, England and Wales, 1847–1982

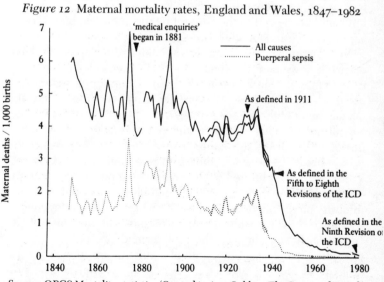

Source: OPCS Mortality statistics (Quoted in Ann Oakley, *The Captured Womb*)

birth position, where, formerly, during hospital childbirth, the woman's legs had been held up and apart in stirrups while she lay flat on her back. Obstetricians (such as Leboyer and Odent) popularised a further childbirth revolution with the introduction into the delivery room of music, chanting, water, and low-level lighting so that the experience of childbirth became a 'ritual of love' and its links with the sexual act were emphasised, a far cry from the surgical act described earlier. The contrast of these two models, one medically dominated, the other consumer-led, is well illustrated in the images present in the 'delivery rooms'.

The battle – for a battle it still is – between who controls childbirth was highlighted by the suspension in 1985 of Wendy Savage, a consultant obstetrician who had espoused the cause of choices in childbirth. She was accused of bad obstetric management in five cases and arraigned in front of a disciplinary enquiry which eventually reinstated her. The case raised all the issues concerning the medicalisation of the birthing process, but in a most graphic way helped to crystallise the opposing models. On one side were senior academic male obstetricians supported by central Health Authority bureaucracy, and on the other a vociferous woman obstetrician supported by consumer organisations, radical midwives and the mothers themselves. The experience was neither gentlemanly nor ladylike for any of the participants, but could be viewed as the attempt by the dominant hierarchy to suppress once and for all the up-and-coming upstart.[17]

Not dissimilar, although less violent, developments have occurred as women, the consumers, have demanded more say in issues ranging from breast-feeding, contraception, abortion, the use of hysterectomies, the premenstrual syndrome and the management of the menopause.

Cultural, sexual, economic and political factors have all influenced the fall and subsequent rise of breast-feeding. Before the 1900s, breast-feeding was the norm in all cultures and classes. Wet-nursing was limited to the nobility and public suckling was accepted. Nevertheless the influence of the rich and powerful minority on the majority resulted in a widespread employment of wet nurses, which only began to diminish at the time of the Industrial Revolution, but they still formed 'one of the conveniences that money can buy', a not dissimilar description of the rise of artificial feeding that occurred post-1900. The medical profession soon began to supervise both the content of milk products and the feeding of infants, but they found themselves at times in opposition to even bigger vested interests. The solution to this 'humiliation' was the unholy alliance of the manufacturer and the medical profession which helped to create the expansion of bottle-feeding.

> The proper authority for establishing rules for substitute feeding should emanate from the medical profession, and not from non-medical capitalists. Yet when we study the history of substitute feeding as it is represented all over the world, the part which the family physician plays, in comparison with numberless patient and proprietory foods administered by the nurses, is a humiliating one, and one which should no longer be tolerated.[18]

The outcome was that breast-feeding was soon to become an exceptional event. In 1923, Mead Johnson could legitimately claim that it was 'responsible in large measure for the advancement of the profession of paediatrics in this country because it brought control of infant feeding under the direction of the medical profession'. The provision of laboratories, research grants and hospital posts funded by manufacturing companies led to a situation where the economic factors rapidly overtook the consideration of either the needs of the baby or the mother so that the same company could write: 'When mothers in America feed their babies by lay advice, the control of your pediatric cases passes out of your hands, Doctor. Our interest in this important phase of medical economics springs, not from any motives of altruism, philanthropy or paternalism, but rather from a spirit of enlightened self-interest and cooperation because (our) infant diet materials are advertised only to you, never to the public.'[19]

Even though comparative studies between bottle-fed and breast-fed babies indicated the dangers of the former, bottle-feeding soon became the norm. The emphasis on the breast as an exclusive sexual organ has helped to influence women's attitudes towards breast-feeding which is seen to 'disfigure' and produce sagging. Paradoxically it is the erotic nature of breast-feeding and its link to sexuality that has influenced its gradual return amongst middle-class women in the last twenty years. Again cultural factors are influential so that in certain societies women's sexual attractiveness is not necessarily linked to full, firm breasts and breast-feeding does not conflict with her image as a sexual woman.

Indeed in Papua New Guinea a dreaded curse is one that will make a woman's breasts stay pert and upright like a prepubertal girl.

The gradual reinstatement of breast-feeding like that of natural birth has resulted from a few pioneering individuals, the rise of consumer organisations and the gradual change in society's perception so that, although 'breast is best' is now more widely accepted, the vested interests in controlling the economics of the product ensure that the battle continues. Nowhere is this more clearly seen than in the baby food industry and Third World nutritional needs. A public outcry and a series of lawsuits against Nestlé's widespread promotion of artificial feeding in Third World countries led to the establishment of a WHO/UNICEF code on the marketing of breast milk substitutes. In summary this code suggests that the following good practice should be observed.

WHO/UNICEF Code

1 No advertising of breastmilk substitutes
2 No free samples to mothers
3 No promotion of products through health care facilities
4 No company mothercraft nurses to advise mothers
5 No gifts or personal samples to health workers
6 No words or pictures idealising artificial feeding, including pictures of infants, on the labels of the products
7 Information to health workers should be scientific and factual
8 All information on artificial feeding, including the labels, should explain the benefits of breastfeeding and the costs and hazards associated with artificial feeding
9 Unsuitable products, such as sweetened condensed milk, should not be promoted for babies

It is because the issue of breast-feeding versus bottle involves such large profits that the medical and social factors have been marginalised by the economic and political ones.[20]

Other areas of health care not specifically related to gender and reproduction, where attitudes towards women have helped to shape the medical approach, include mental health care (chapter 12) and the treatment of obesity.

In the same way that the medical profession took control over women's reproductive systems and the multi-national companies took control over bottle-feeding, the fashion and food industry has literally helped to shape the size and form of women's bodies. One needs only to contrast the 'ideal' shape of women's bodies in the Sixties as depicted by Twiggy, an exceptionally slight fashion model, to that painted by Rubens in the seventeenth century, to recognise that this is yet another area where women have accepted a mode of being in their bodies which importantly affects their health. Being overweight, anorexia nervosa, bulimia and compulsive eating disorders are far more prevalent amongst women, and have been medicalised in the same way as pregnancy and infant-feeding were a century earlier. Food and its preparation is in almost all cultures the traditional province for women: woman's place has traditionally been in the kitchen, preparing food for others, whether it is the school break, sandwiches for lunch or the Sunday dinner. At the same time Western culture's obsession with slimness emphasises that fatness is an unhealthy sign which requires treatment by dieting. A multi-million pound industry, involving women's magazines, the food industry, health clubs and diet books, has developed to ensure that the inevitable double-bind in the message to women is maintained, i.e. you are responsible for your family's food, but you cannot eat too much lest you become overweight and fat.

It is not surprising that this coercive message has been challenged by the feminist movement and that books like *Fat is a Feminist Issue* and the 'Women's therapy centre for eating disorders' have appeared in the last fifteen years.[21] They are the equivalent of the Natural Childbirth and Breast is Best movements. They illustrate how the medical construction of women as patients stems from cultural and societal views of women and women's bodies. As women are beginning to achieve more equal status in society and the rigid cultural norms are breaking down, medicine has had to redefine its definition of pathology and treatments. In the same way as the feminist movement influenced society's attitudes towads nuclear warfare through its much publicised campaign at Greenham Common, so it has begun to shape medical approaches to the understanding of women, health and illness.

It has been argued that the dominant medical ideology of women as 'frail beings' helped to confirm two requirements. Women are 'too weak' to become doctors and can only fill the role of 'patients'.[22] These attitudes are still fairly prevalent today and comments such as these are not uncommon.

There is only moderate enthusiasm in the medical profession for an increase in the number of women doctors. [23]

I always worry about families where the wife and mother is a doctor. I cannot see how a woman can lead such a life and at the same time be a wife to her husband and more importantly, a mother to her children. [24]

This is at a time when nearly 50 per cent of medical students are women and women outnumber men in training schemes in general practice.

The power relationships between men and women still dominate the practice of medicine and as Ehrenreich and English write:

Medical science has been one of the most powerful sources of sexist ideology in our culture. Justifications for sexual discrimination – in education, in jobs, in public life – must ultimately rest on the one thing that differentiates women from men: their bodies. Theories of male superiority ultimately rest on biology.

Medicine stands between biology and social policy, between the 'mysterious' world of the laboratory and everyday life. [25]

Thus although there have been many changes within the discipline of medicine the shift in attitudes sought by many feminists is still a long way away. In addition, medicine and the other health-care professions have experienced some of the consequences that are associated with the militant feminist movement. For instance, it has been argued by some that the vulgar attitudes of dirty, dishevelled women did more harm to the anti-nuclear cause than to promote it. Furthermore it is difficult to see how the encouragement of antagonism, hostility, harsh and unloving attitudes can be considered part of any health-care approach. Nevertheless it is as a result of the emergence of the 'feminine principle' as opposed to feminism that many important changes are occurring within medicine. The principle culturally associated with the attributes and skills of listening, nurturing, containing, receptiveness, has led to the introduction of the therapeutic interventions of touching, massage, relaxation, meditation, as well as a recognition of the importance of communication skills in health care. The 'greening process' has helped to identify the importance and necessity of these attributes not only to us as individuals but to our social institutions. In articulating this dimension, some individual women have had to shout to be heard. Their 'extremism' needs to be seen within the context of the 'masculine' bias so clearly prevalent both within medical care and our culture.

10

The Dignifying of Death

In the *Tibetan Book of the Dead*, which is a treatise on 'how to die', it is considered that it is not possible to judge the value of a person's life until one has witnessed his manner of dying.[1] The Trukese, a Micronesian society, consider that the process of dying begins at forty. When a Trukese reaches the age of forty he can no longer climb trees as well as he used to, his strength begins to wane and when that happens he begins to prepare for his death.

Much of our own culture is geared not only to denying death but to retarding the ageing process. Science and medicine have lent themselves readily to this process. We have developed an impressive array of procedures, chemical agents, multivitamins, mineral preparations, and reconstructive surgical processes whose aim is to prolong life, often at the expense of living. Once patients were removed from home so that they could die in hospital, we limited our contact as well as our children's with death. That is not to deny that hospitals and expert nursing do not

Table 8 Total deaths and percentage of deaths occurring in non-psychiatric hospitals (NHS and other) and at home, in selected years between 1965 and 1979, England and Wales

	All deaths (England and Wales)			All neoplastic disease		
		Non-psychiatric hospitals –			Non-psychiatric hospitals –	
Year	Total (1000s)	NHS and other (%)	Home (%)	Total (1000s)	NHS and other (%)	Home (%)
1965	549	50	38	107	60	37
1970	575	54	33	117	61.5	33
1974	585	56	31	123	64	31
1979	593	57	29	130	64	30

play a valuable part in caring for the terminally ill patient. Indeed it could be argued that more suffering occurred at home than in hospital and several surveys by the Marie Curie Foundation (1952)[2] and Hinton[3] seem to suggest that romanticising the death-bed scene at home is a real danger. Although traditional cultures may well have responded to death differently from us, psychologically death has always been a fearful and frightening experience.

Probably there is no greater factor which determines the nature of our health-care system than our attitudes towards death. Much of medicine is organised and devoted to do battle with death. Doctors and nurses consider themselves to have failed if a patient dies. Studies amongst doctors have found them to be afraid of death in greater proportion than a control group of patients[4] and a time-and-motion study of a hospital ward indicated that doctors and nurses spend less time with a patient once they have identified that he is dying.[5] These attitudes coincide at a time when the percentage of people dying in hospital is continuing to increase. It is against this background that several remarkable pioneers began their work which has helped to influence not only our attitudes towards the terminally ill but our approach to patient care in general.

Early Indian cultures in America would shoot arrows in the air to drive away the evil spirits associated with the dead. Firing guns at military funerals is not too dissimilar a ritual. Because of his fear of death and his inability to 'know' the answers to the perennial question 'Is there life after death?', man has tended to deny the existence of this inevitable event and erect a complicated edifice of subterfuge and evasion which permeates the topic. Nevertheless, it is possible to trace certain consistent patterns of behaviour and forms of belief which are present in many different cultures. Rituals are seen as 'rites of passage', the only accepted forms of behaviour which surround a naturally occurring human and social transition, e.g. birth, marriage, death. In his examination of rituals surrounding death, Hertz[6] observed that two forms of death are commonly observed: biological and social death. Between these two events a period of time elapses which may be a few days to a year or indeed may be prolonged for ever. Biological death is the loss of physical identity – the person's body is no longer present, and social death is the loss of the person's presence-influence and enables the family to continue living without him. The transition between biological death and social death is that period when living members help the dead to enter the 'land of his ancestors'. It can be a dangerous period for everyone and is often marked with prescribed forms of dress – the wearing of a black dress for widows in many countries. The period of shib'ab amongst the Jewish community lasts precisely one week; mourning dress is worn for thirty days, and amusement is forbidden for one year. Many Mediterranean women wear black continually after their husbands' death. In many cultures a widowed woman is considered to be like her husband, suspended between life and death. By and large Western societies' view of death has largely been influenced by the three great religions of Christianity, Judaism and Islam. We are indebted to Socrates for a very detailed view of the dying process during his dialogue with his friends Simmion and Cebes and faithfully recorded by Plato. This particular dialogue occurred on the day Socrates took poison, so his views are not only theoretical but were influenced by his knowledge of his impending death.

Socrates felt that philosophy – the love of wisdom – was 'simply and solely the practice of dying – the practice of death', and to deny this meant that the individual was not a philosopher. Socrates' view of the body is very similar to that found in Eastern texts – a prison. Death provided the opportunity for the soul to travel to its rightful destination – God – and he felt each person had a guardian spirit which helped guide the soul once released back to Hades. This journey was difficult and had many 'breaks and branches' and entailed the crossing of many rivers – Acheron – the river of pain, Pyriphlegthon – the river of burning.[7]

Judaism has three great tenets – free will, God and immortality – and like Socrates believes that death sets the soul free and permits it to depart the mortal life. When Rabbi Bunam was dying, his wife was weeping unconsolably by his side. 'Why weep?' he said, 'All my life has been given me merely that I might learn to die.'

Christianity teaches that the human soul is not naturally immortal. Only through Christ's resurrection and belief in that can the soul reach Heaven, 'He that believeth hath eternal life'. Unlike many Eastern religions, Christianity does not believe in destiny or fate. Through the act of forgiveness and atonement, Grace enters the human being and his journey to God is assured – body and soul. For many people, both Eastern and Western, the concepts of resurrection and reincarnation, although very different, provide the hope that dispels the fear of death. Death in all the major religions has involved a meeting with the Gods whether 'Natural' or 'Divine'. Indeed Greek doctors under the influence of Hippocrates believed it to be unethical to treat a patient who is in the grip of a 'fatal illness', for to do so, the doctor pitted himself against nature and ran the risk of that fateful hubris that awaited those mortals who challenged the Gods.

In the seventeenth century the process of dying was a leisurely affair attended by much visitation. Several diaries of the time have recorded such visits. Philip Aries, in his book *The Hour of Our Death*,[8] describes the 'good death' in Europe as one where order was created both in spiritual and temporal terms. In all these descriptions we see how different societies attempted to provide some form of structure to the process of dying which allowed for the individual and his family to share an experience which was felt to be inevitable no matter what the cause.

In the nineteenth century, with the increasing influence of medicine, we begin to see a separation between natural death and abnormal death. Natural death was seen to come without previous sickness or obvious cause. It is very rare to find a picture of a doctor or nurse at a death-bed scene before the nineteenth century. After the First World War, pictures depict doctors fighting valiantly against death, tearing a young woman from a skeleton – locking a skeleton in the cupboard. The doctor now begins to stand between us and death. The final chapter in this process is the transformation of our Health Service to a death prevention service, with the doctor standing as umpire in some complicated game determining when and where individuals may join or leave the game.[9] In *The Indignity of Death*[10] Ramsey wrote in 1974: 'There is a growing agreement amongst moralists that death has again to be accepted and all that can be done for the dying is to keep them company in their final moments.'

At about the same time, Elizabeth Kübler-Ross began her multi-disciplinary seminars on the care of the dying patient. Her point of departure was her perception that dying in hospital was lonely, mechanical and dehumanised. Following some major resistance from medical staff, she interviewed over 200 patients who were in the last stages of life. This was the first time that any systematic attempt had been made to obtain the views from patients of this inevitable consequence to terminal disease. Each interview was tape-recorded and analysed. Kübler-Ross's five

'Stages of Dying' are now taught in many different clinical institutions. Although providing a structure for understanding why a
patient may be behaving in a particular way, they can also be used
as yet another checklist of questions, thus avoiding the human
contact that will keep them company in their final moments.
Nevertheless Kübler-Ross's work has allowed for a greater discussion to take place and has begun to break down the taboo
surrounding death amongst health-care workers.

The five 'stages of dying'

1 *Denial* – 'No not me.' This is a typical reaction when a patient
   learns that he or she is terminally ill. Denial is important and
   necessary. It helps cushion the impact of the patient's awareness that death is inevitable.

2 *Rage and anger* – 'Why me?' The patient resents the fact that
   others will remain healthy and alive while he or she must die.
   God is a special target for anger, since He is regarded as
   imposing, arbitrarily, the death sentence. To those who are
   shocked at her claim that such anger is not only permissible but
   inevitable, Doctor Ross replies succinctly 'God can take it'.

3 *Bargaining* – 'Yes me, but . . .' Patients accept the fact of death
   but strike bargains for more time. Mostly they bargain with God
   – 'even among people who never talked with God before'. They
   promise to be good or to do something in exchange for another
   week or month or year of life. Notes Dr Ross: 'What they
   promise is totally irrelevant, because they don't keep their
   promises anyway.'

4 *Depression* – 'Yes me.' First, the person mourns past losses,
   things not done, wrongs committed. But then he or she enters a
   state of 'preparatory grief', getting ready for the arrival of
   death. The patient grows quiet, doesn't want visitors. 'When a
   dying patient doesn't want to see you any more', says Dr Ross,
   'this is a sign he has finished his unfinished business with you,
   and it is a blessing. He can now let go peacefully.'[1]

5 *Acceptance* – 'My time is very close now and it's all right.' Dr
   Ross describes this final stage as 'not a happy stage, but neither
   is it unhappy. It's devoid of feelings but it's not resignation, it's
   really a victory.'[11]

The Hospice Movement

The hospice movement grew out of a realisation by its pioneering
founder, Dame Cicely Saunders, of the inadequacies and difficulties encountered by patients, their relatives, doctors and staff
when caring for the terminally ill within NHS hospitals. In 1869
over 80 per cent of deaths occurred in people under sixty-five; in
1969 this figure is 30 per cent. Less than a tenth of people dying in
1869 died in institutions, whereas this figure now is approaching
70 per cent. In addition, over a fifth of all deaths are now due to
cancer of some kind or another. The conclusion to draw from these
figures is that death is more concentrated amongst the elderly,
and is more associated with chronic illness and prolonged care.
Two extensive surveys identify both the needs and attitudes of the
terminally ill and the responses both clinical and personal of the
medical services.[12] Inadequate levels of funding, support services
and personnel are part of the reason why the hospice movement
has grown as rapidly as it has.

   Under Christian influence, the care of the dying patient began
to assume more than just medical care. St Luke's Hospice (1893)
and St Joseph's Hospice (1905) were early examples of the
modern-day equivalent and themselves were the continuation of
mediaeval monastic medical orders and the deaconess hospitals of
Europe. St Christopher's Hospice was founded in 1967 with the
express intention of not only providing terminal care for the
in-patients but developing an education and research centre to
enable other practitioners to learn the principles of terminal care.
At a recent international symposium (1989), representatives from
all over the world gave strong evidence to the growth of this
development in our health-care services. Under the guidance of
Dame Cicely, the philosophy of terminal care has slowly evolved
and its influence had a far wider impact on the caring of patients in
general. A nun in St Joseph's Hospice expressed one of the
guidelines offered to all medical and nursing personnel: 'Feelings
are facts in this house', and the concept of 'total pain' – physical,
mental, social and spiritual – was introduced to widen people's
horizons concerning the nature of the task required of the medical
staff.[13] It became clear that many doctors and nurses experienced
difficulty in talking to dying patients. Few people seem to be able
to talk to dying patients with ease. In hospital the culture is
generally one of denial both amongst doctors and relatives. 'Don't

tell, he will give up hope', 'It is cruel to tell him he is going to die' are not uncommon responses, and the subsequent automatic prescribing of antidepressants or tranquillisers is an understandable if inappropriate consequence. Fear of being blamed or expressing emotion or unleashing a reaction are coupled with fear of not knowing all the answers and, above all, of having failed to keep the patient alive. If the central goal of medical care is seen to be that of preventing death, then the doctor and staff responsible for the dying patient will find it impossible to avoid these commonly held fears, and they will inevitably colour his or her responses to patients' questions. In numerous surveys the strengths and difficulties encountered by both doctor and patient in discussing the subject of death reveal that this is far more a cultural difficulty than a specifically medical one. Saunders points out that the provision of a containing environment can often reduce the level of anxiety and fear that prevents adequate communication. This containing environment applies equally to staff as well as to patients, and one of the important developments coming from the hospice movement has been the realisation of how essential this component is. Staff support groups are now found in other settings where the demands of the patient are both psychological and physical. Frequent meetings with all staff members including ward orderlies, students and consultants, help to reduce anxiety and allow for the expression of painful and inadequate feelings amongst individual members. The care of the dying has helped to recognise that total patient care does not require total individual involvement – indeed this may be to the detriment of both patient and staff member. A further feature of the hospice movement has been its emphasis on family involvement and a flexible home-care policy. The boundaries between in-patient care and home-care have purposely been kept fluid, and several hospice and palliative care units now have a home-care support team who visit the patient at home and liaise with existing community services. In addition an impressive expertise has developed regarding the management and control of symptoms in terminal care. All too often in the past the dying patient was left unattended, with the misguided view that 'nothing could be done'. Nevertheless a recent survey (Table 9) suggests that much still needs to be done to help the professionals concerned acquire the necessary expertise to make the time around death 'an indefinable atmosphere which [leaves] one feeling that death [is]

Table 9 The symptoms of terminal illness according to the average of reports from relative, hospital nurse and GP (percentages of 262 cases, in numerical order)

Symptom	Total	Uncontrolled
Pain	52	35
Weakness	52	50
Dyspnoea (difficulty in breathing)	42	35
Immobility	41	39
Urinary incontinence	35	16
Anorexia	32	30
Anxiety	24	22
Cough	24	21
Confusion	23	21
Vomiting	20	16
Bowel problems (other than incontinence)	19	14
Insomnia	19	16
Depression	18	17
Nausea	16	10
Faecal incontinence	13	12
Dysphagia (difficulty in swallowing)	10	10
Pressure sores	9	6
Offensive odours	5	5

Source: Wilkes, P., *A Source Book on Terminal Care* (University of Sheffield).

nothing to be worried about – a sort of coming home'.[14] A list of helpful attitudes for patients and their families (Table 10) indicates how open and hopeful the care of the dying has become.[15]

Bereavement and grief

At the same time as an understanding of the need of the dying patient developed, it became clear that the survivors required the help of the health-care professionals. Dying of a 'broken heart' and 'grief' was not an uncommon cause of death in the seventeenth and eighteenth centuries. More recent studies have indicated quite how at risk the survivors are.

Parkes' classic work amongst widows and widowers showed an increased mortality rate in the first six months following the death of their spouses. More recently this has been linked to changes within the immune system of the survivors.[16] A further study showed an increased mortality in the first year of bereavement

Table 10 Make today count

Helpful attitudes for terminally ill persons and their families

1 TALK about the illness. If it is cancer, call it cancer. Don't try to hide what is wrong.
2 ACCEPT DEATH AS A PART OF LIFE. It is.
3 CONSIDER each day as another day of life, a gift from God, to be enjoyed as fully as possible, rather than another day closer to death.
4 REALIZE that life is never going to be perfect. It wasn't before and it won't be now.
5 PRAY; don't be ashamed or afraid. It isn't a sign of weakness . . . it is your strength.
6 LEARN to live with your illness instead of considering yourself dying from it. We all are dying in some manner.
7 PUT your friends and relatives at ease yourself. If you don't want pity, don't ask for it.
8 MAKE all practical arrangements for the future and make certain your family understands them.
9 SET new goals: realise your limitations. Sometimes the simple things of life become the most enjoyable.
10 DISCUSS problems with your family as they occur. Include the children, if possible. After all, your problem is not an individual one.

and concluded that this risk was present amongst other close relatives and not just the surviving spouses. The rate of divorce amongst parents of children dying of cancer is 80 per cent and the preventive value of bereavement counselling to high-risk groups using the 'key person' card developed at St Christopher's Hospice illustrates how sensitive and well-constructed research can aid in the appropriate use of the counselling services.[17]

Guides on the psychological reaction to the loss of a loved one have helped identify the various responses that are commonly found. Parkes (1972) describes a process of realisation which may go through different stages: (a) shock, disbelief, denial, followed by (b) an intense preoccupation and longing for the lost person, moving through (c) a period of depression, dejection and hopelessness, with finally, (d) a period of acceptance and resolution. Over a period of five years, six relatives of patients who died at St Christopher's committed suicide, and it is clear that working with the survivors can be as difficult and as daunting a task as working with the patients. Feelings of anger and guilt are common and need to be acknowledged and allowed for. Psycho-analytic studies of the mourning process have further strengthened the view that the acceptance of the sadness associated with any loss is a very necessary part of the maturative development of the human species – 'All change involves a loss and loss needs to be mourned'. In a similar manner that working with the dying patient has enhanced the understanding of patient care in general, working with bereavement and grief has enabled patients and clinicians to understand the necessary psychological and emotional work that may require to occur following other losses – e.g. termination of pregnancy, removal of a breast, amputation of a limb, loss of potency following a heart attack, etc. The consequences of many such occurrences that bring people into hospital are all associated with important and emotional reactions. The physical recovery process is influenced, to some degree, by the appropriate responses that are encouraged by the professional staff. Similarly, all 'rites of passage' are linked to the potential for gain as well as the experience of loss. Counselling the unemployed or the recently retired executive, broken relationships as well as broken marriages require an understanding that the mourning process forms part of our normal human experience and is not solely to be associated with the loss of some close relative.

These developments in the care of human beings have encouraged and allowed for the expression of feelings so that the management of death is not seen as a technological and medical failure. Indeed, it can be an opportunity for the exchange of what is now accepted as fairly healthy behaviour. Our definition of health begins to alter once we allow for the importance of these human experiences. The impact of these changes on the professional care worker has been immense. No longer is it acceptable to communicate 'about' the patient at the end of the bed without communicating 'with' the patient. The advice to remain distant and objective and not get involved is no longer valid if one is to undertake emotional work of any kind. It is a disturbing business and will often affect and, at times, overwhelm the individual involved. The level of appropriate distance and appropriate intimacy may need to be discovered with each patient, and there is a clear requirement to provide adequate supervision and staff support groups for individuals involved in working with patients who make demands of this nature.

At first glance it may be difficult to link the changes described in

Figure 13 'Key Person Card'

<table>
<tr><td></td><td>CONFIDENTIAL</td><td>Case Note</td></tr>
<tr><td>Name of patient</td><td>Age</td><td>Number:</td></tr>
<tr><td>(surname first in capitals)</td><td></td><td></td></tr>
<tr><td></td><td>Date of admission</td><td>Date of death</td></tr>
</table>

Surname of key person Address:

First Name:

Telephone

Relationship to patient   O.P. Yes/No

Do you think key person would object to follow up?   Yes/No/Not known

Staff members(s) most closely involved:

Other family members in need of help:

Comments (include details of help already being given):

FSP   Signed: p.t.o

Questionnaire (Ring one item in each section. Leave blank if not known: CONFIDENTIAL

...... Tick here if key person not well enough known to enable these questions to be answered.

A.	B.	C.	D.	E.
Children under 14 at home	**Occupation of principal wage earner of key person's family****	**Employment of K.P. outside home**	**Clinging or pining**	**Anger**
0. None	1. Profs. & Exec.	0. Works FT	1. Never	1. None (or normal)
1. One	2. Semi-profes.	1. Works PT	2. Seldom	2. Mild irritation
2. Two	3. Office & clerical	3. Retired	3. Moderate	3. Moderate occasional outburs
3. Three	4. Skilled manual	4. Housewife only	4. Frequent	4. Severe spoiling relationships
4. Four	5. Semi-skilled manual	5. Unemployed	5. Constant	5. Extreme always bitter
5. Five or more	6. Unskilled manual		6. Constant intense	
	** If in doubt, guess			

F.	G.	H.
Self-reproach	**Relationship now**	**How will key person cope?***
1. None	0. Close intimate relat. with another	1. **Well.** Normal grief and recovery without special help
2. Mild vague and general	2. Warm supportive family permitting expression of feeling	2. **Fair,** probably get by without special help
3. Moderate—some clear self-reproach	3. Family supportive but live at distance	3. **Doubtful,** may need special help.
4. Severe—preoc. self blame	4. Doubtful	4. **Badly,** requires special help.
5. Extreme—major problem	5. None of these	5. **Very badly,** requires urgent help.
		* All scoring 4–5 on H will be followed up.

Source: C. Saunders, *The Management of Terminal Malignant Disease* (1984).

caring for the dying with the Green movement. The latter has arisen in part out of the recognition of the ecological links between animate and inanimate matter, the survival of one species with the survival of another. Ecology which lays claim to 'fundamental biological notions' has much to say regarding the nature of change within the universe and the links between life and death. It has been observed that human beings can be certain of two things only: that change will occur, and that death is inevitable. It would seem sensible therefore that medicine, which itself lays claim to the science of life, should address these two consistent features of our lives. As the practice of medicine begins to incorporate some of the thinking found in ecological texts regarding the nature of change and death, then we can expect to see the pioneering work described in this chapter having more influence on the daily work of doctors and other health-care practitioners.

11

The Gentler Way with Cancer

If the nineteenth-century disease was tuberculosis, then the twentieth-century disease is cancer. There are nearly 250,000 new cases of cancer each year and it is estimated that one in three people will suffer from cancer at one time during their life. The word cancer itself has become a stumbling-block for a proper discussion of the subject and the stigma attached to having cancer can cause more distress and suffering than the disease itself. The word cancer conjures up thoughts of pain, emaciation and death. It is used as a 'catch-all' word to describe some of the most lethal diseases as well as some that can be classified almost as a normal part of the ageing process. Skin cancer is curable in 98 per cent of all cases and cannot be compared to lung cancer where only 7 per cent of patients will survive five years.[1] The use of the label 'cancer' can be compared to the use of the label 'fever' in the nineteenth century. Doctors would diagnose one as having a 'fever' no matter whether it arose from a minor infection or a serious condition such as typhoid. Part of the fear that surrounds cancer can only begin to be allayed when some of these mistaken perceptions are addressed.

When fear predominates our responses to a particular situation, then we seek powerful allies and protectors to shield us from the feared object. The word 'growth', often used with the word 'tumour' as a synonym for cancer, suggests an understandable response by both patient and doctor – 'take it out'. If there is an abnormal growth that should not be there, then removal should effect a cure and prevent recurrence. This commonsense response has guided what is often the first line of treatment – that of surgical removal.

Although surgery is clearly appropriate in many situations, it is now thought that by the time a cancer has grown large enough to be detected either by examination (breast lump) or X-ray (lung), the tumour cells will have been growing for several years and that spread is likely to have occurred elsewhere. Even though surgical removal may not effect a total removal it will reduce symptoms and prolong life. However, the nature of the surgery offered has now changed and this is most clearly obvious in breast cancer. There was a time when some surgeons advocated the removal of both breasts in case cancer developed at some future date in the 'normal' breast. Radical mastectomy was the routine approach offered to all breast cancer patients up until two decades ago. This involved the removal not only of the breast but of all the muscles of the chest wall and glands in the armpit. The unfortunate woman was left with a gross disfigurement and the likelihood of a swollen and painful arm on the side of the operation, due to the removal of all lymph drainage. In 1972 the relevance of surgery to long-term survival was challenged[2] and further studies indicated that, although the removal of the breast resulted in a decrease in the local spread of the disease, it did not reduce distant metastases. It is now possible to offer women several alternatives regarding the surgical treatment of breast cancer. Lumpectomy (the removal of the lump with minimal surrounding tissue) has increasingly become the norm. Although surgery and anaesthesia are that much safer now than they were twenty or fifty years ago, many women are requesting to know the biopsy result first before deciding on whether to proceed with surgery. In the past surgeons would remove the growth, have it analysed, and remove the breast, all during the same operation, so that permission had to be given by the patient before she was aware of the precise nature of the growth.

Surgery is increasingly being used for the control of symptoms in cancer patients and its place as a curative intervention has been reassessed. Together with the reduction of gross surgery has come a reappraisal of the other two forms of orthodox treatment for cancer, radiotherapy and chemotherapy. The rise in the incidence of some cancers (skin cancer and leukaemia) has been related to increased levels of radiation, either as a result of some nuclear disaster (Chernobyl) or the destruction of the ozone layer.

Radiotherapy

Radiotherapy, a form of reversed homoeopathy, kills growing tissue and has been successfully used as the treatment of choice for several cancers. Two methods of delivering radio-active material are employed, either by focusing radio-active radiation from an external source on to the tumour, or by implanting or injecting radio-active material directly into the cancerous tissue. The effects of radiotherapy depend on the *frequency* and amount of radiation required to kill the cells and the depth to which the radiation travels within the body. When this form of therapy was first used, the local effects of radiotherapy were particularly unpleasant, but more refined calculations and machinery have made this particular problem more manageable. However, the more general side-effects which amount to a form of radiation sickness can be most troublesome and unpleasant.

Symptoms can include tiredness, nausea, los of appetite, vomiting, diarrhoea and depression. Tiredness is by far the most common symptom, followed by nausea. Both can be alleviated by drugs and many patients find that proper information before the radiotherapy, together with some relaxation and breathing techniques, helps to prevent these general symptoms. Many radiotherapy centres now employ counsellors to ensure that patients are adequately supported during this course of treatment. The severity of the 'general symptoms' will depend partly on the patient's general level of well-being (diet, exercise, relaxation, etc.) and partly on the frequency and dose of radiation. Radiotherapy applied to the head, neck and limbs does not produce as severe symptoms as when applied to the trunk and abdomen. Like surgery, radiotherapy can be used to treat the terminal stages of cancer to relieve distressing and painful symptoms, even if it does not actually prolong life. Radiotherapy will often completely remove all cancer cells (cancer of the cervix) and avoid having to undertake unnecessary surgery. Both surgery and radiotherapy have nevertheless been overused and oversold as a form of treatment in cancer.

Chemotherapy

Many patients fear the use of drugs to treat cancer. Again, this can be founded on a misunderstanding of the nature of cancer. In some cancers, chemotherapy is the treatment of choice and the response can be excellent. Twenty years ago, leukaemia in children was almost invariably fatal. Now many children survive and are cured simply with chemotherapy. Chemotherapy is often used as a second or third treatment when the cancer has spread and surgery or radiotherapy is no longer appropriate or possible. It is on these occasions that there is a justified need to apply caution, as the results of chemotherapy in disseminated cancer are doubtful and temporary at best. The side-effects of chemotherapy are usually more general and more severe than either surgery or radiotherapy. Cancers where chemotherapy is very useful are:

- Hodgkin's disease
- Leukaemias
- Testicular tumours
- Multiple myeloma
- Wilms' tumour (in children)
- Choriocarcinoma

Chemotherapy is the name given to drugs which attack growing cells. They were first discovered after the First World War when the effect of mustard-gas was discovered – it caused a reduction of white cells. It was decided to give a form of nitrogen-mustard to patients with leukaemia (a blood cancer where white cells proliferate). There are now over fifty drugs which have been used for treating cancer and the greatest success has occurred where drugs are given in combination as a 'cocktail'. Some drugs can be taken by mouth, others require the patient to be admitted to hospital and the drug is injected into a vein or passed through a drip-feed. These drugs act generally by interfering with the growth of cells, either by combining with the DNA (gene that controls growth of cell), or by blocking the production of the necessary ingredients required for cells to multiply (anti-folic acid drugs). Recently it has been possible to develop drugs which attack only the cancer cells and thus the side-effects and problems related to chemotherapy are reduced. Side-effects of chemo-therapy are:

- Nausea, vomiting
- Stomatitis
- Loss of hair
- Sterility
- Diarrhoea
- Low blood count
- Bone-marrow depression
- Skin rash
- Local pain if injected outside vein

Nevertheless, chemotherapy can be an unpleasant form of treatment. The most distressing, although the least serious of the side-effects, has been the loss of hair that almost always accompanies chemotherapy. If warned ahead of the time, the patient can obtain a suitable wig, which will allow for some psychological comfort. The hair almost always grows back again once the treatment is ended. The general symptoms of nausea, vomiting, stomatitis and diarrhoea can often be countered by the appropriate use of anti-emetic, kaolin, vitamin and mineral supplements. The more serious side-effects, which include the lowering of the blood count and the development of secondary infections, require frequent blood tests to ensure that the white cells do not fall below a certain level. Bleeding and bruising may also occur if the 'platelets' are damaged.

It is against this background that the growth in alternative approaches to cancer management has arisen. Cassileth[3] has argued that such alternative or complementary therapies are functions of the social climate in which they exist, both taking shape out of and affecting that climate. They are based on the 'Rambo approach' to medicine in which losing the fight against cancer becomes a personal weakness. Their popularity is based on the fact that cancer symbolises the limitations and uncertainties within medicine. These limitations and uncertainties have resulted in attempts to control and overcome the cancer or growth. Surgery, radiotherapy and chemotherapy can be seen as symbolising the aggressive 'masculine' response to 'being out of control'. There is nothing inherently wrong with adopting an aggressive approach *per se*, and indeed we have seen how the results in certain cancers are excellent. However, for the majority of cancers, these approaches have not substantially affected patients' long-term survival, and they have undoubtedly caused a diminution in the quality of life of cancer sufferers.

Thus the aspects that seem to attract patients to the newer therapies are often based around a more holistic approach to patient care.[4] It must be emphasised, however, that it is certainly not the case that all complementary therapies are holistic in their outlook, or that all, or even many, doctors are not holistic in their approach to patient care. The things that patients are looking for are varied and diverse. In many people's minds cancer is often associated with a slow, painful death.[5] A healthy approach to death can often dispel much anxiety, and accepting that death is not a failure, that one can be healed spiritually and yet die physically, and allowing the patient to 'die well' by paying attention to the details of dying can often make an enormous difference to the patient.[6] The treatment of cancer patients has drawn very heavily on the work described in the previous chapter. Another characteristic of many complementary therapies is that they give some measure of control back to the patient, allowing him or her to regain self-esteem. Supposedly simple skills such as listening to the patient, or massage and touch can be very beneficial.[7] It is often the case that the patient chooses the therapist and not the therapy, that is to say that he or she is more interested in finding someone with whom a good professional relationship can be established than in the particular therapy.[8]

Some medical commentators have appreciated the failure of the medical profession to provide what amounts to the hallmarks of 'good medicine', sympathetic and supportive care for their patients, during a very stressful time, especially when the medical treatment is often perceived as worse than the disease. They have suggested that the medical profession learn from their mistake.[9] It has been suggested that such support groups be set up within the hospitals treating cancer patients.

In the last few years this has indeed occurred within both the orthodox and alternative fields. The Bristol Cancer Help Centre, which was opened by Prince Charles in 1983, arose out of the experience of one of its founder members once she herself had developed breast cancer. The principles underlying the work of the clinic have slowly evolved and include:

1 Holistic approach – responding to patients' physical, emotional, psychological and spiritual needs
2 Patients have the right to assume some responsibility for their own health
3 Teaching and practising life-style changes to prevent cancer occurring and recurring
4 Use of 'safe and gentle' therapies to counteract disease and enhance life.

The initial response from patients was immediate and the clinic soon found itself overwhelmed with demands both nationally and internationally. There was much resistance from the medical profession to the claims made for cures and even greater concern when patients refused orthodox treatment to pursue the therapies advocated at Bristol. Such therapies are often based around simple or intuitive ideas about disease. Often a belief in the ability of the mind to affect the body is found.[10] They tend to be long-term and associated with a change in life-style.[11] Diet often plays a crucial role,[12] and a spiritual aspect is commonly found.[13] Often such therapies cause little or no harm, and being involved in them is of great benefit to patients,[14] but there is a more sinister side to be considered. Some therapies are based on pseudo-science, and are anti-medicine, rejecting any invasive procedure, even if it is of proven benefit.[15] There are certainly charlatans who play on the need of the patient with cancer in order to make money;[16] some would say up to 10 per cent of complementary therapists are like this. As a result, and because of certain well known, but probably ineffective therapies, there have been re-peated calls from within the medical profession for doctors to have nothing to do with complementary therapy in the treatment of cancer.[17] Usually objections from the medical profession arise from the lack of objective scientific data showing such therapies to be of benefit, although it is not always easy for complementary therapies, often based on non-Western ideas of causality and treatment of disease, to conduct trials which meet the rigorous requirements of the now accepted randomised, controlled clinical trial. In this situation the cry of 'quackery' is never far from the lips of the established medical profession. Again we can see how many of the issues described earlier – the use of power, inter-professional collaboration, the nature of scientific evidence – all come together in the controversy surrounding the treatment of cancer.

Nevertheless collaboration between orthodox systems and complementary systems is beginning to occur and the necessary research into the claims made for some of the therapies has suggested that not all can be dismissed as quackery. Indeed, several of the orthodox centres of excellence in the treatment of cancer have begun to incorporate some of the principles of management pioneered by the Bristol Cancer Help Centre. The two most important areas of exploration have been the importance of psychosocial and dietary factors in both the causation and management of cancer.

Psychosocial factors

In one, a prospective, controlled study of over 1,000 men, those who later developed cancer scored significantly worse on a 'closeness to parents' scale (fewer positive attitudes, more negative attitudes than healthy groups). This was not the case for groups who subsequently developed essential hypertension, or coronary heart disease.[18] When analysed this was found to be a measurement of self-reported father/son relationships. Its association was still significant after adjustment for a variety of known risk factors (such as smoking) was made.[19] Mental attitudes have also been linked with cancer.[20] Of smokers, those who get lung cancer tend to be less self-assertive than those who do not.[21] A less well-balanced approach to interpersonal relationships, ambivalent attitudes towards life, and fewer intellectual interests have also been linked with cancer.[22] The important question is whether this is a causal link. The circumstantial evidence linking psychological correlates to cancer is becoming too great to dismiss lightly.[23] It has been suggested that the link is neither indirect (i.e. by association with another independent risk factor) nor direct, but the link is probably a concomitant of the associated disease state (i.e. it is a real link, but not a causal link). It just happens that people who are likely to get cancer have this tendency towards poor parental relationships.[24] On the other hand, it is also possible that psychological factors are merely one link in the chain of causation, operating in a continuum of somatic disease, with more effect on cancer and less effect on coronary heart disease.[25] Some have argued that the idea of psychological causation leads to blame being ascribed to the patients for his or her disease, and so to a feeling of guilt.[26]

The idea that stress is one of the causative factors in the development of cancer is still not yet accepted by orthodox medicine. The various relaxation, meditation and visualisation techniques now utilised as a way to 'love your cancer away' together with the supportive psychotherapeutic approaches form part of the accepted 'gentle' models of cancer therapy. The techniques challenge the materialist base to bio-medicine and suggest that mental states can influence the workings of the immune system with respect to its effect on the progression of a cancer. There is some evidence to support these precepts.[27]

The therapy which has received the most public interest is

perhaps the Simonton technique of guided imagery. The patient is encouraged to imagine his white blood cells eating/destroying the cancer cells in his body. Alternatively a symbolic representation can be used. In this way the common view of cancer as a powerful and destructive disease is turned around. The cancer cells are described as 'weak' and 'confused', whilst the body's immune cells are described as 'strong' and 'powerful', like sharks attacking meat. It is claimed that this enhances the body's immune system, increasing its ability to detect and destroy tumour cells. The Simonton programme includes group therapy to help resolve the underlying problems associated with cancer, and to help to develop coping skills. This may be one reason why they have found it difficult to establish which part of their programme is of the most benefit. There has been no conclusive proof that this therapy can produce significant tumour regression. A prospective randomised controlled trial did show that less aggressive imagery could produce significant improvements in the mood of patients with breast cancer undergoing treatment.[28]

Dietary factors

There has always been good epidemiological evidence relating dietary fibre and colorectal cancer. Fibre is known to bind carcinogens (cancer forming residues) and reduces intestinal transit time by a factor of two. Seventh-Day Adventists, whose diet is mostly lacto-vegetarian, and therefore contains much dietary fibre, have a much lower incidence of cancer compared to the average American.

Known constituents in the diet such as mycotoxins and nitrosamines have been implicated in carcinogenic experimental studies on animals. Similarly, low levels of dietary fat, and an increase in vitamin C, vitamin E, retinoids, and flavinoids have all been shown to protect against experimental cancer. Human studies have linked cancer to poor intake of vitamin A and carotenoids.

Other interesting findings are that blood selenium levels are generally depressed in patients who have cancer and that people who have a very low level of blood selenium have double the risk of developing cancer overall.[29]

The diet therapies share a common philosophy: poor diet can help cause cancer, and so a good diet can help cure it. Some therapies aim to rid the body of toxins that accumulate from the food we tend to eat in the Western world, by such means as fasting or eating only fruit. Common principles found amongst the dietary therapies are strict vegan or vegetarian adherence, large amounts of raw foods, sugar free and low in salt, the use of vegetable/fruit/liver juices and high doses of vitamins/minerals/enzymes.[30] However, it has been argued that the diets generally used in dietary therapies are exactly the opposite of the needs of most cancer patients.[31] They are high in bulk and low in calories, often unpalatable, difficult to prepare and costly to follow. The usual outcome is weight loss, weakness, depression (if the diet is not enjoyable), guilt (if the patient has to stop the diet), and anger (if the diet produces no result).[32]

It is clear that the debate regarding complementary approaches to cancer will continue for years but the aggressive masculine therapies associated with orthodox medicine – surgery, radiotherapy and chemotherapy – are slowly being challenged and complemented by the use of psychotherapy, mental imagery and dietary interventions, examples of 'gentler' and more 'feminine' approaches. Here again the consumer has been at the forefront of these changes. The rapid growth and success of the Bristol Centre and self-help organisation, e.g. BACUP (British Association of Cancer United Patients), suggest that yet again, patients may be leading the medical profession into areas of care it has either neglected or derided.

12

The Managing of Misery

'Most men (and more women) live lives of quiet desperation.' The form this desperation takes will vary from individual to individual and from culture to culture. The language used to describe human behaviour, which is viewed as outside normal parameters, will reflect the belief system prevalent at the time, and the response to the 'abnormal' individual will be dependent on numerous factors least of which is the understanding of the nature of mental illness. Stafford-Clark, in his excellent review *Psychiatry Today*,[1] quotes Gregory Zilboorg, the medical historian:

> Every mental patient either aggressively rejects life as we like it
> – and he was therefore thought of as heretic, witch, or sorcerer –
> or passively succumbs to his inability to accept life as we see it
> and he was therefore called bewitched.[2]

People with mental illness have over the years been burnt at the stake, tortured, incarcerated, scapegoated, drugged, lobotomised and psycho-analysed, to name only a few of the interventions that have been used. The study of the mind and its workings has developed slowly and the causal undertaking of mental illness is still very much in its infancy.

For many primitive peoples the mind and the soul were inseparable concepts and, as the soul was subject to the forces present in nature through the power of the Gods, man's mind was at the mercy of being taken over by the Gods. Cultures with rigid rules regarding normal and abnormal behaviour developed rites and ceremonies where inverted or abnormal behaviour was permitted and socially catered for. Festivals and carnivals, Mardi Gras, Halloween, April Fool's Day are ritualised ceremonies where abnormal, 'mad' or 'inverted' behaviour by individuals or groups was countenanced and formed part of the yearly calendar. Individuals dressed in strange clothes either with direct reference to animals and nature or the spirits and the Gods. They were given licence to act differently and outrageously. When 'abnormal behaviour' occurred outside these ritualised ceremonies, society's response varied. For some, being 'possessed' was viewed as a 'gift' and seen as normal: no attempt to re-train or punish the individual occurred. However, for the majority of Western and 'civilised' countries, the responses were not so accepting. For several centuries, the persecution of the 'possessed' was viewed as a religious duty: 'Thou shalt not suffer a witch to live'(Exodus XXII, 18), 'A man also or woman that hath a familiar spirit or that is a wizard shall surely be put to death – they shall stone them with stones, their blood shall be upon them' (Leviticus XX, 27). Notwithstanding the Bible's admonitions and Christ's own casting out of the devils, the early church maintained its hold on the mind, insisting that mind and spirit and soul were all closely linked and thus fell within the province of the authority of the clergy.

That the mind is linked to the brain is a relatively recent idea. The Ancient Egyptians believed the mind-spirit-soul resided in the bowels and the heart. The Sumerians thought it resided in the liver. Aristotle believed the heart was the centre for thought and feeling. Plato did not believe in trusting the senses and arrived as his description of the mind through a mixture of mystical contemplation and mathematics. Because he valued reason above all other attributes, it followed that the mind should reside in the topmost part of the body, the head. Both Aristotle and Plato were instrumental in seeing the mind's chief faculty as reason and logic, and the early Christian church incorporated some aspects of their philosophy. The early church had a major incentive for maintaining the notion that mind, spirit and soul were all closely linked. This not only gave the church leaders control over the study of the mind, but allowed the church to dictate what the mind should think, feel and imagine. The persecution of witches and the tortures during the Inquisition were justified because the victims of these activities showed obvious signs of deranged minds. For the church, a healthy and sound mind meant believing in and following the dogma prescribed by the church. An unhealthy mind and abnormal behaviour indicated a refusal to accept the authority of the church and an alliance with the forces of evil.

Psychological disturbance was not seen as the special province of the physician, and even Hippocrates, whose observation on mental illness broke fresh ground, found the whole weight of public opinion against him. Hippocrates tried to establish the study of mental illness based on observation and not on philosophical descriptions and mystical meditation. He recognised the importance of the brain as the organ of the mind – he enumerated a system of physiological explanations for disorders of mood and temperament and he denied that the Gods had anything to do with illness. He attempted to rescue the disease of epilepsy from the label of 'Sacred Disease'. He considered this condition 'in no way more divine, or more sacred than other diseases but having a natural cause'. By studying the brains of epileptics he believed 'You will see that it is not a god which injures the body but disease'. He believed that people using the idea that epilepsy was a divine disease 'used divinity as a screen for their own inability to offer any assistance'. Hippocrates' view of epilepsy and mental illness did not gain ground and the persecution and incarceration of the mentally ill continued. About the middle of the first century BC, another Greek physician, Asclepiades, denounced the use of the cells and dungeons used to restrict such patients. In what appears to be a thoroughly modern treatise, he suggested that mental illness resulted from emotional conflict and that rest, warm baths, comfortable beds, music, harmony and pleasant company were required to restore mental peace. Soranus, a pupil of Asclepiades, continued his work and it is possible to discern in his writings debates which are still relevant today:

They prescribe placing all patients in darkness . . . without ascertaining whether or not this measure adds another burden . . . rather than being themselves disposed to cure their patients, they seem to be in a state of delirium; they compare their patients to ferocious beasts whom they would subdue by deprivation of food and the torments of thirst. Misled no doubt by this error they advise that patients be cruelly chained, forgetting that their limbs might be injured or broken and that it is more suitable and much easier to restrain the sick by the hands of men than by the weights of often harmful iron. They even advise bodily violence, like the use of the whip, as if such measures could force a return to reason; such treatment is deplorable and only aggravates the patient's condition; it stains the body and limbs with blood – a sad spectacle indeed for the patient to contemplate when he regains his senses.

Soranus advocated an approach which can be viewed as a remark-able document on the treatment of the mentally sick, but unfortu-nately not one that was pursued with any vigour:

> If any part of the body has suffered from the patient's restless-ness warm applications, held by soft and very clean material to the head, shoulders, and chest, are useful. It is necessary to employ fomentations of mixed warm oil, a light decoction of tallow or of linseed oil being preferred because of its softening qualities. Frequent comings and goings, especially on the part of strangers, should be forbidden, and the attendants should be rigorously advised to limit the excursions of the patients so that they will never be exasperated by too much vivacity. Neverthe-less, it is equally necessary to avoid increasing their unreason-ableness by too much activity and resulting feebleness.
>
> Much tact and discretion should be employed in directing attention to their faults; sometimes misbehaviour should be overlooked or met with indulgence; at other times it requires a slightly bitter reprimand and an explanation of the advantages derived from proper conduct.

The period from 200 AD, immediately following Asclepiades, right up until the eighteenth century saw the return of the theory of demonology as a cause of mental illness and the church held sway over their treatment. The first recorded execution of a witch occurred around 430 AD, and over the next twelve centuries, hundreds of thousands were persecuted and killed. Pope Inno-cent VII issued a Bill in 1484 empowering 'supreme inquisitors' to examine and try the heretical so that Christianity might be purged of the invasion by 'demons, witches, succubi, incubi and other similar forces'. The *Malleus Maleficarum* (The Hammer of Witches) is the mediaeval treatise by which abnormal behaviour on the part of the mentally sick was to be recognised and exting-uished. It has been described as a 'volume so insane, so cruel and leading to such horrible conclusions that never before or since did such a combination of horrible characteristics flow from human pen'. By the fourteenth century most towns in Europe had a secure cell or dungeon where the insane could be forcibly de-tained. The Tollhaus, the Tollviste (mad cell) and the Tollkobein (mad hut) were the precursors of the asylums and mental hos-pitals. Individuals did attempt to stand against the view as expressed in the *Malleus Maleficarum* but were either themselves accused of demonology or banished from professional life.

It was not until 1736 that the laws against witchcraft were repealed, and not until the last quarter of the nineteenth century that the medical profession assumed full responsibility for the care of the mentally ill.

Before then, Samuel Tuke, a philanthropist, Quaker and social reformer introduced 'The Retreat'. In a report to his committee he wrote:

> There were not any day rooms with contiguous airing courts. There were but two airing courts for all the classes of patients, except the opulent, who took their exercise in the garden. All the other classes of men were turned into one court, and the women into the other. There was no provision in either court for shelter against the rain or heat. Very few of the patients were allowed hats, and shoes and stockings were not unfrequently wanting. In this state, you might see more than 100 poor creatures shut up together, unattended and uninspected by any one; the lowest paupers and persons of respectable habits, the melancholic and the manic, the calm and the restless, the convalescent, and the incurable. It is needless, and it would be painful, to enumerate the evils and the dangers resulting from this system of indiscriminate association. The danger of patients injuring each other was also very great, from their being shut up in considerable numbers in their day rooms, without any attendant or inspector.[3]

There was concern regarding the contagiousness of what was termed 'prison fever' and many of Tuke's reforms were concerned with the reduction of these infections. Leprosy, the disease of the fifteenth and the sixteenth centuries, had diminished in its importance, and the 'prison hospital' replaced the Lazar House. Tuke's reforms focused on a more individualised approach to treatment as well as replacing punishment and coercion with hygiene and education. He proposed warm baths and human kindness and was highly critical of the medical treatment of the insane.

At about the same time Phillipe Pinel became physician superintendent of the Bicêtre Hospital in Paris. He instituted changes not dissimilar to Tuke – inmates were unchained; blood-letting,

Table 11 County asylums in England and Wales

	Asylums	Patients	Average no. patients
1827	9	1046	116
1850	24	7140	297
1860	41	15845	386
1870	50	27109	542
1900	77	77004	961

Source: Bryan Turner, *Medical Power and Social Knowledge* (1987) Sage.

ducking and every form of violence were abolished. He introduced a system of dietary management and ventilation which reduced the incidence of gaol fever.

Thus the development of psychiatry proceeded along two different pathways. On the one hand, 'authorities' had to respond to the need and seemingly increasing number of 'insane'. On the other hand, individual physicians and psychiatrists developed theories and models of the mind which allowed for the introduction and development of newer therapies. By the nineteenth century there was a steady increase in the number of asylums (Table 11). These often housed the paupers and vagrants found in an increasingly industrialised society. Several Parliamentary Reports drew attention to the insanitary conditions, and as successful cures were rare, the population of such institutions grew. Society had little option but to adopt a 'warehouse' approach to the treatment of the mentally ill. However, by the beginning of the nineteenth century, studies of the mind became more common and the influence of mesmerism and hypnosis was particularly strong. Charcot, the brilliant French neurologist, established this form of therapy at the Salpetrière Hospital in Paris. His brilliance was renowned and he made use of this form of therapy to differentiate between paralysis caused by organic disease and that caused by hysteria. However, even Charcot's observations were to prove to be incorrect and it was his young student Freud who was to herald a new development in the study of the insane. Charcot was unable to demonstrate abnormalities on autopsies of women patients who had been diagnosed as hysterical. Freud left Paris and returned to Vienna to develop his own theory of hysteria which was based on the idea that the patient's mind was not scarred by organic lesions but by unconscious forces. Freud's genius has rightfully gone unchallenged. Some of his earlier theories on sexuality may have reflected the problems of Viennese society and have attracted criticism, as has the use of psycho-analysis as a therapeutic modality. Freud's greatest gift to the study of mental illness was to give importance to the patient's own responses. Thus doctors, psychiatrists and mental welfare workers began to understand the importance of 'listening to the patient'. No longer was the patient to be the object of study – he was to form part of the study himself. It has taken many years since Freud for the patient with mental illness to be afforded the privilege of being listened to.

The study of psychiatry, like physical medicine, was revolutionised with the development of pharmacological and physical interventions which developed at the same time as Freud was undertaking his own studies. With the development of powerful psycho-active drugs, a new chapter in the history of psychiatry began. Drugs which affected levels of arousal and mood were prescribed as sedatives and formed the basis of the development of the modern tranquilliser. Anti-confusion or anti-psychotic drugs such as Largactil (phenothiazine) found a place in the treatment and management of schizophrenia and other psychotic conditions. A further group of drugs were the anti-depressants used to elevate mood and treat depression which was increasingly viewed as the result of a chemical imbalance within the brain.

By the 1970s, psycho-active drugs became the second most commonly prescribed group of drugs, and it was estimated that, in one night in seven, sleep is aided by either a tranquilliser or sleeping tablet. This increase in medication seemed not to reduce the level of psychiatric morbidity in the population. In 1983 6 per cent of all new out-patient referrals were for psychiatric conditions and 52 per cent of all hospital beds were for psychiatric disorders – 42 per cent of those patients in psychiatric hospitals had been in-patients for longer than five years.[4] It would seem that one of the major results of the psycho-active drug approach to the treatment of mental illness was that the less disturbed patients were discharged from hospital and managed in the community. Between 1959 and 1980 occupied psychiatric beds were reduced by one half. Thus, although there were no fewer psychiatric patients, and indeed the figures suggested an increase in psychiatric morbidity, more were being managed in the community than in hospital.

The Sixties saw the discipline of psychiatry under attack from several prominent figures. Goffmann's critique of mental asylums, although not new, drew attention to the state of such institutions in the same way as Tuke and Pinel had done previously.[5] Thomas Szasz in his condemnation of the medicalisation of mental illness prepared the ground for the leader of the anti-psychiatry movement, R. D. Laing.[6] Laing became one of the persistent critics of the medical model and his radical reappraisal of what constitutes mental illness was seen as challenging the political, cultural and economic norms of acceptable behaviour.[7] Laing's theories of mental illness were not dissimilar to the sociological analysis of mental health which has been referred to as *social reaction theory* or *labelling theory*. This theoretical position suggests that deviant behaviour is defined and determined by the powerful, influential and dominant social groups in society. The nature of deviant behaviour, mental illness and forms of madness is based more on the socially accepted norms than on some consistent and objective illness. This approach to mental illness suggests that once someone is labelled 'mad', he or she will suffer stigmatisation which will accentuate his sense of alienation and thus formalise his 'illness' into a life-long career of 'madness'. In addition, attempts by social agencies either through psychiatrists, social workers and mental hospitals are all doomed to fail because, by and large, they all accept and conform to the dominant mode of behaviour.[8] In support of this hypothesis of 'social labelling' Rosenheim examined and described the outcome of what happened when nine professional and academic people feigned mental illness and presented themselves to psychiatric out-patients complaining of hearing voices. Eight were diagnosed (labelled) as schizophrenic and all nine as manic depressive. They remained undetected by the medical staff although some patients were able to correctly identify their pretence.[9] Labelling theory received much support in the Sixties and Seventies, and together with Laing's critique led to a reappraisal of the biological base to mental illness. Partly as a result of this reappraisal, many of the mental hospital patients were discharged into the community.

This shift from institutional care to community care, although heralded as an advance in the management of mental illness, has given rise to much criticism. Families have been unable to reintegrate their disturbed relatives. The lack of social provision, community support and adequate accommodation has resulted in many of these unfortunate patients swelling the ranks of the vagrant population of our inner cities. Worse still, there has been an almost identical increase in the prison population which reflects the decrease in the numbers of psychiatric inmates. No adequate research has been undertaken to explore the possible link between these two alterations but much anecdotal evidence supports the view that many of our prisons now house the former inmates of our psychiatric institutions.

A further development of the social-labelling theory of mental illness occurred as the result of the understanding derived from adopting the 'life events' model. This model proposed initially by Meyer but developed by other workers suggested that mental illness occurred at points where individuals were exposed to and experiencing social stresses whilst being separated from their usual support systems.[10] Mental illness has always been more frequently diagnosed in women and the incidence of depression is twice as high in women as in men. Brown, using the life events model, identified a series of social circumstances (unemployment, presence of pre-school children, lack of a close intimate friend) which predisposed to a sense of hopelessness, low self-esteem and depression.[11] This study, amongst many others, forced the psychiatric professions on the defensive. Not only was organic psychiatry, with its use of powerful drugs and physical therapies (ECT), under attack, but so was the very basis of psychiatric illness as a disease with organic and biochemical aetiologies.

It was not surprising therefore that the focus for many involved in psychological work moved away from illness and pathology to growth and health. The Sixties and Seventies saw a vast expansion of what has become known as the 'new psychotherapies'. Psychoanalysis, with its emphasis on the unconscious and the shadow side of human nature, was replaced by humanistic models of psychological understanding. This school drew its theoretical framework from the existential philosophers and the Gestalt psychologists. Humanistic psychologists, of whom Maslow was the foremost, emphasised the need for creativity, self-expression and self-actualisation. The focus of these therapies was to encourage and maximise the potential that lay within each of us. Therapists trained in these methods emphasised the strength of the conscious mind and its ability to overcome unconscious forces. Positive thinking was encouraged and the client was directed to living in the 'here and now' rather than the past or future. A feature of many of these new therapies is that they were 'client-centred'.

Carl Rogers, one of the original founders of this movement in psychotherapy, strove to move away from the medical model, not only in its theoretical formulation but in its practical application. He felt that the psycho-analytic method as developed by Freud maintained the therapist in a powerful position within the transaction. He emphasised the need for the client to take charge of the psychotherapeutic exchange and underlined the need for the therapist to remain non-directive.[12] The term psychotherapy became ambiguous and misused. The egalitarian nature of the new psychotherapies included a demystification and an attack on the need for 'professional training'. Carefully conducted outcome studies seemed to indicate that similar results could be achieved by psychotherapists of different persuasions, no matter what their length of training.[13] Indeed, one study suggested that managers, trainers and academic tutors who would not normally describe themselves as psychotherapists, obtained equally good results as the professionals. A further study suggested that the attributes of the therapist him or herself were more important in determining the outcome than the type or length of training. These attributes, genuineness, warmth, transparency, could be found with equal frequency in untrained psychotherapists as much as in trained psychotherapists.[14]

More recently, these new psychotherapies have themselves come under criticism, not so much for the methods they use but for the underlying assumption – that perfection is possible within one lifetime – and that to achieve this state of wholeness is everyone's right and destiny. Nevertheless, these basic assumptions have been very influential in America and increasingly so in the United Kingdom. The growth movement has spawned hundreds of different therapies, each searching for the elusive 'self' and each determined to be 'authentic' and offer the correct path towards enlightenment.

Meanwhile the needs of the mentally sick continue to grow. The confusion that surrounds the practice of psychiatry, both organic and psychotherapeutic, is as great as it was in previous centuries. We have seen in turn the rise and fall of the mental asylums. The hope that psycho-active drugs would finally allow psychiatry to work on a rational and biochemical basis disappeared as the ingestion of millions of tranquillisers and sleeping tablets failed to provide the answer. Psycho-analysis and psychother-apies, both new and old, seemed to offer a gentler and more humane solution to the miseries besetting the population. Many people have avoided institutional mental care as a result of the 'talking cures' but the demand for counselling and psychotherapy appears to be immense. These therapies seem to offer help and support during vulnerable and stressful points in people's lives but the total number of psychiatric patients has not decreased and if anything has increased.

The dilemma faced by psychiatry can be expressed in terms relevant to the Green movement. How do we as a society deal with what is difficult, alien and uncomfortable? How do we deal with that which is no longer wanted or useful, be it our household rubbish, an out-of-date car or a mentally disturbed relative? If as individuals we expect 'the Government' or 'the psychiatric com-munity' to create systems to manage those rejected aspects of our lives, then we may find that the solutions they adopt will eventu-ally lead to an ecologically unbalanced state of affairs. For no government, however popular or creative, can forever deal with our individual rubbish, and no group of mental health-care pro-fessionals, however skilled, can continue to protect us from the responsibilities we have to carry for being mentally healthy. These responsibilities necessitate the sharing of the misery so many of the less fortunate members of our society experience. The management of this misery requires a process of sharing so that the muddle and confusion that abounds in the discipline of psychiatry may be the price we have to pay for a more tolerant and flexible approach to the problems of our inner minds. The crisis that is overwhelming the discipline of psychiatry has coincided with the emergence of several consumer movements for the protection of the mentally sick (MIND, MENCAP). Again, we see an example of the greening process within medicine, i.e. the acceptance of limits, the sharing of power, the demystification of the professional expert, and the emergence of the consumer interest group.

13

The Return of the Spirit

Man's initial attempts at understanding the workings of the universe entailed creating a panoply of Gods and Goddesses. These powerful figures of his imagination controlled the wind, the sea, the sun and all other aspects of his environment with which he came in contact. Man felt his insignificance in relation to the Gods and erected a whole edifice of belief and practice to enable him to communicate effectively with these powerful forces. Witch-doctors, shamans, priests were selected by man to become the mediators between him and the Gods. Elaborate rituals, sacrifices, incantations, ceremonies were developed as a means of both appeasing the Gods as well as demanding their favour, blessings and recovery from illness. The shaman or tribal religious leader is found in almost all cultures and is the *primogenitor* of all subsequent health-care practitioners. He combined the roles of both priest, doctor and social worker, and the religious nature of healing ceremonies formed an essential part of the ritual of health care. The shaman would enter into a trance either through the drinking of some hallucinogenic herb or after the performance of a repetitive chant or dance. Whilst in the trance he would engage with the evil spirits or offer sacrifices to the God who had been offended.

The illness that had entered the patient was seen to have been caused by some spiritual transgression, and it was only through the mediation of the priest/shaman that the illness could be transformed and the patient regain his health. The magical quality of the ritual was often accompanied by empiric interventions – drugs, herbs, poultices, enemas and physical manipulations. Study of the details of these empiric interventions suggest that the shamans were astute physicians as well as magicians. Nevertheless, the early history of medicine and healing is linked strongly to the belief that man's spirit or soul formed an integral part of his being. Illness and health were inextricably linked to his spiritual nature and that powerful external forces directly determined the course of his life and death. The organised churches whether Jewish, Christian, Islam or Hindu were all concerned with health and healing and several of the earliest 'medical' textbooks are to be found in the great scriptures of the day. It was not only the religious leaders who were involved in determining the appropriate healing practices. Hippocrates is seen as having laid the foundation of modern Western medicine. But the three great philosophers who preceded him and followed each other – Socrates, Plato and Aristotle – all involved themselves in matters medical, and taught on the appropriate relationship between doctor and patient. Much of the early discourses between Plato and Aristotle describe and delineate the difference between phylo-techne (love of the art) and phylo-anthropos (love of the man). These two attributes guided the doctor in his approach to his patient. Hippocrates, who is seen as having inspired and collated the body of works that bears his name, helped to introduce an element of objectivity and empiricism in medicine. Nevertheless he was a firm believer, like Plato before him, that

> The cure of the part should not be attempted without treatment of the whole. No attempt should be made to cure the body without the soul and if the head and body are to be healthy you must begin by curing the mind, for this is the greatest error of our day in the treatment of the human body that physicians first separate the soul from the body . . .[1]

The mediaeval Christian church held firmly to the belief espoused by Plato and continued to exercise its power over doctors. The mediaeval practice of 'trial by ordeal' implied that as long as the soul was pure no harm could be done to the body even if it were plunged into boiling oil or burning brazier. With the advent of the earliest medical schools in Italy and France, the church still maintained a strong hold on the study of anatomy. Dissection of bodies was forbidden.

Thus the early church had a major influence in maintaining that mind, spirit and soul were all closely linked and helped determine the functioning of the body. This not only gave the church control over the study of the mind and body but allowed it to impose guidelines as to what the mind was allowed to think, feel and imagine. For the early church, a healthy mind meant believing in its dogma and an unhealthy mind meant allying oneself with the forces of evil.

As I have already pointed out, the explosion that occurred during the Renaissance heralded a major shift in medicine as in all other areas. Copernicus, Galileo, Descartes, and Newton all helped to propel the study of man away from the narrow dictates of the church and towards the rational and scientific model that has held sway for the last three hundred years. This process of secularisation led to a division of the patient. The care of the soul became the legitimate focus for the church and its priests whilst the study of the mind and body was acknowledged as the basis of future medical developments. The spirit or soul with its immaterial and unknowable qualities became more and more difficult to incorporate within the developing framework of scientific medicine. Indeed it seemed as if the mind was also to be excluded from the proper study of medicine and it is not until the latter part of the nineteenth century that attempts to study the mind were made with any earnestness. We need only remind ourselves of the difficulty psychiatry has had as a discipline in establishing itself as a legitimate specialty in medicine to appreciate how much a problem the reintegration of 'the spirit' into the study of medicine may well prove to be. Precise definitions and clear statements regarding the spirit do not come easily. For many it is difficult to separate spirit from mind. Yet all the scriptures of whatever religion imply that the spirit is more than the sum of emotional and psychological states. The divide between spirit and mind is not helped by the fact that the translators of Freud translated the German word *der Siele* (soul) as 'mind' and used the Greek word 'psyche', meaning soul, to describe mental structure. Thus, in a cosmic Freudian slip, the discussion regarding the separation between mind and spirit is made almost impossible, and the language available only helps to perpetuate the confusion. Table 12 gives some of the more popular definitions of spirit.

The *OED* gives 'spirit' four pages and twenty-four sub-sections including 'the animating or vital principles in man', 'the soul of a person as commended to God', 'active or essential principle or power of some emotion or state of mind', 'subtle or intangible element or principle in material things'. It may still not be clear from these definitions how the spirit of a person is separate from his mental state and the nearest it may be possible to arrive at for a convinced materialist is that the spirit like the wind is a force you cannot see but which you know by its effects. In Christian terms the spirit has always had some association with death or rather life after death. The strong Christian belief in life after death came from its very beginning – the resurrection of Christ – and for many it is soul or spirit that lives on after death. It is this transcendent quality that helps to differentiate spirit from mind. It is seen, though not always, to involve a consideration of something greater than oneself. It is often associated with an experience, a sense of harmony or peace – a knowing from within, and many spiritual practices endeavour to encourage the development of these experiences.

Another possible method of arriving at a definition of spirit that can begin to be integrated within a materialistic and causal world view is to examine the spiritual practices and interventions associated with priests', Rabbis' or Shamans' work and place them alongside possible similar interventions found in more secular settings. A comparison such as outlined in Table 13 may suggest that the idea that the general practitioner has taken over the role of the priest is not so far-fetched as it may seem. A brief description of a few of those interventions outlined will emphasise the difficulty of separating spiritual interventions from psychological and physical ones.

Sanctuary/safe space

Churches were built not only as places of worship but to serve as sanctuaries from invading forces. They were seen as protected territory providing the itinerant traveller with shelter and warmth. Spence describes the unit of medical practice as 'the occasion when in the intimacy of the consulting room a person

Table 12 What is Spirit?

• Immaterial part of man	• Inspired
• Religion/beliefs/conviction	• Emotional calmness
• Soul – vitality	• Everyday ecstasy
• Quintessence of various forms	• Sense of harmony
• Life force	• Sense of belonging
• Breath of life	• Knowing sure from within
• A possession	• Transcendent force
• Something higher	• Mystical experience

Source: P. C. Pietroni, 'Spirited Interventions in a General Practice Setting' (1986) in *Holistic Medicine*, 1, 253–262.

Table 13 The role of priest and role of general practitioner

Spiritual practice	General practice counterpart
1. Providing a sanctuary	Consulting room as a 'safe space'
2. Confessional	Active listening
3. Interpret tribulation	Give meaning to stressful life events
4. Source of ritual and ceremony	Repeat prescription
5. Provide support and comfort	Teamwork
6. Increase spiritual awareness	Give permission for spiritual discussion
7. Laying on of hands	Use of touch
Prayer and meditation	Relaxation and quiet time
8. Communion	Self-help groups/patient participation

Source: P. C. Pietroni, 'Spiritual Interventions in a General Practice Setting'.

who is ill or believes himself to be ill seeks the advice of a doctor whom he trusts'. The words 'intimacy' and 'trust' invoke the notion of the consulting room as a 'sanctuary' or safe space. Fry, in his book *Safe Space*, traces the use of this concept in medical settings and draws attention to the importance of architecture and colour in conveying an atmosphere where healing can be enhanced.[2]

Confessional/active listening

The act of unburdening oneself of troubled thoughts, feelings, resentments is an act as old as man himself. It formed part of all spiritual traditions: 'Give up what thou hast and then thy will receive' is translated in more popular words as 'Confession is good for the soul'. Since the notion of sin as a cause for distress has been replaced by the notion of repression, the drama has moved from the confessional to the analytic couch, psychotherapist's chair or general practitioner's consulting room. The Greek word 'catharsis' or 'cleansing' is seen as the first stage of the psychotherapeutic process and Jung writes: 'The goal of the cathartic method is full confessional – not merely the intellectual recognition of the facts with the head, but their confirmation by the heart and the actual release of suppressed emotions.'[3] Many of the psychotherapeutic techniques developed in the first half of this century to aid the process of confessional, from free association to hypnosis and breathing exercises, have similar counterparts in shamanistic practices and, as pointed out by Sargant, are not dissimilar to the brainwashing techniques found in interrogation and counter-intelligence centres.[4] However, it is the emphasis on active listening within the consultation between doctor and patient that has been emphasised in clinical text-books and the following advice is to be found in a text-book titled *Six Minutes for the Patient*. It is important for the doctor to free himself from trying to discover *why* so that he can observe *how* the patient talks, thinks, feels and behaves the way he does.'[5] The psycho-analyst who inspired this piece of research never mentioned the word spirit or soul once in his writings, yet he could write:

> The aim of all human striving is to establish or probably re-establish an all-embracing harmony with one's environment – to be able to leave in peace. The 'union-mystica' the re-establishment of the harmonious inter-penetrating mix-up between the individual and the most important parts of his environment his love objects is the desire of all humanity.[6]

The phrase 'harmonious inter-penetrating mix-up' strikes a chord with many spiritual descriptions of the true nature of man.

Laying on of hands/use of touch

Touching, laying on of hands and blessings have always formed part of spiritual practice and is validated within the Christian church from references to the scriptures. Christ in direct instruction to his disciples as described in Matthew (10.8) – Heal the sick, raise the dead, cleanse the lepers, cast out devils. For St Luke Jesus healed through touch – 'the power of the body'. European royalty, who claimed to rule by divine right, took on this power and by 1307 the public in need of healing were visiting Philip the Fair, the King of France. The English kings soon followed and touching for tuberculosis became a common practice; the condition became known as the King's Evil, and the royal touch and laying on of hands formed part of the accepted practice of spiritual healing. In 1600 one practitioner was so successful he became known as 'the stroker'. The claims made by many of these itinerant healers were challenged forcefully, much as today, so that Thackeray in his book (of 1841), *Extraordinary Popular Delusion and the Madness of Crowds*, wrote how 'Mr. Valentine Greatraks practised upon himself and others a deception that God had given him the power of curing the King's Evil'. Nevertheless the laying on of hands still remains the most popular of all spiritual interven-

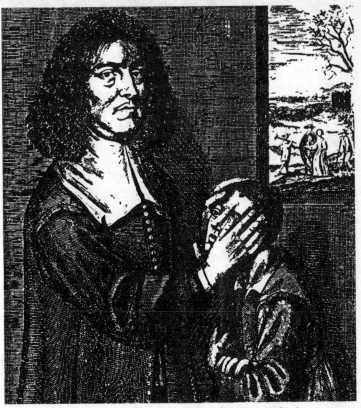

Figure 14 Valentine Greatraks, the 'Stroker'

tions, and the scientific community has very reluctantly studied
its secular equivalent of touch with some trepidation. Montagu
points out, citing many examples from animal and human behaviour, how the skin and touching form an essential psychological and physiological first step in the proper development of the
other sensory systems of the body.[7] Deprivation dwarfism is a
well-recognised condition that occurs in institutions where children, in spite of good food and medical care, fail to thrive because
they are not held, touched and hugged.

Licking for some animals plays a very important role in maternal behaviour and is likened to patting and stroking of the human
baby. Similar activities such as oiling, preening, head scratching,
dusting and sunbathing have their counterpart in human behaviour. Hammett in 1922 stumbled on the beneficial effects of

touch, when he was investigating the effects of electric shocks on rats. One group of rats was put in a cage and subjected to electric shocks. A second group was put in a cage and left there. The third group was left in the nest. It was the second group which was left alone and not handled that did worst by all parameters.[8] Harlow's classic experiments with baby monkeys carry this work one step further. A baby monkey was put in a cage with two models – one made out of wire and one out of soft cloth. The one with wire provided milk and food. When the monkey was stressed it ran to the model made out of cloth and spent most of the time clinging to the soft surrogate mother. Harlow concluded that contact comfort was a more important source of mother-child relationship than food-source comfort.[9] Studies of babies and infants do not differ in their findings, namely that touch and body contact is an essential factor in the physical, mental and emotional development from a very early age.

More recently in its survey on *Alternative Therapy*, the BMA committee identified the use of touch as one of the contributory factors for the popularity of many such therapies.[10] Spiritual healers in an attempt both to quantify and validate the 'laying on of hands', or therapeutic touch, have conducted several experiments both with inanimate material, plants, human beings and complex electronic equipment. Several clinical trials are currently under progress, testing the claim that therapeutic touch will limit the growth of cataracts and eradicate intestinal parasites in horses.[11] Notwithstanding the claims made for therapeutic efficacy, the use of touch, massage, holding, laying on of hands etc. has increased in clinical and secular settings and in the most recent survey of alternative practitioners in the UK the largest group were found to be spiritual healers.[12]

Prayer and contemplation/relaxation and meditation

As outlined earlier, one of the ways in which 'spirit' has been interpreted is to separate it altogether from organised religion and a set of beliefs and link it to a 'special way of being'. Spirit and spiritual states are seen as something beyond the mundane and everyday. The notion of spirit is linked to the concept of life-force, a transcendent or mystical state of consciousness. It is this link to consciousness that has produced a reawakening of interest and study into matters spiritual. Like spirit, consciousness can be difficult to define but we can come nearer to studying and observing different states of consciousness through the use of electro-encephalograms and the measurement of brainwave activity. The very many disciplines that have been involved in the study of consciousness have all arrived at a different definition:

By consciousness I understand the relation of psychic contents to the ego in so far as this relation is perceived as such by the ego. Relations to the ego that are not perceived as such are unconscious. Consciousness is the function or activity which maintains the relation of psychic contents to the ego.

Jung

A fact without parallel which defies all explanation or description. Nevertheless if anyone speaks of consciousness we know immediately and from our most personal experience what is meant by it.

Freud

Consciousness is the recognition of the fact that there is an inner being who knows what is real and who is in charge of the organism and what happens.

Philip Lee

Our normal waking consciousness, rational consciousness, as we call it, is but one special type of consciousness, whilst all about it, parted from it by the flimsiest of screens, there lie potential forms of consciousness, entirely different. No account of the universe in its totality can be final which leaves these other forms of consciousness quite disregarded.

William James

Consciousness is 'that of which one is aware'.

Psychologists

Ordinary consciousness is an exquisitely evolved personal construction – sensory systems select a small amount of input data, the brain modifies and gates this sensory input; higher level cortical selectivity filters on the basis of needs, preconceptions and 'sets'.

Ornstein

Ordinary consciousness is an illusion.

Hindu text

According to which assumptions we make, the stream of consciousness is one of the following:

1 a complex of mental activities changing and flowing in time;

2 a succession of states, each real yet different in quality and
   kind from each other;
3 a personal participation in universal (cosmic) consciousness;
4 a flow of personal experience;
5 an epiphenomenal by-product of continuous brain functioning;
6 a matter of schedules of reinforcement provided by our social
   environment;
7 subjective awareness correlated with brain functioning;
8 a set of emergent properties or characteristics.

J. Strange

It is the link with 'special states of consciousness' and the
spiritual practices of prayer, meditation, contemplation, that have
drawn millions of people back to some form of 'spiritual practice'.
And it is the assumed link with positive health, a 'sense of well
being', 'inner peace', 'harmony', 'balance' that has seen the
growth of the consciousness therapies. By transforming one's
consciousness it is believed that unwanted, unpleasant and unhealthy aspects of behaviour and emotions can be altered. Nearly
all of the newer psychotherapies – mind-body therapies and
humanistic therapies, work on the assumption that healing involves an alteration in consciousness and the development of
awareness. 'Becoming aware' and 'maximising one's potential' are
the buzz words of the growth movement that arose during the
Sixties, and that form part of modern secular spiritual practice. It
is easy to dismiss many of these approaches to health-care as signs
of the narcissistic-culture and self-absorption linked to Western
affluence. However, the end-point to many of these practices
appears to be remarkably similar, and secular descriptions of
these states of consciousness are almost identical to those found
in Buddhist, Christian and Jewish literature. They have been
described by poets and writers throughout time. They have in
common elements which lift them out of ordinary emotional
experiences one may have on a day-to-day basis. Their extraordi-
nariness is often startling and for many may mark the beginning of
profound changes, psychological as well as physical.

> . . . that serene and blessed mood
> In which the affections gently lead us on –
> Until, the breath of this corporeal frame
> And even the motion of our human blood
> Almost suspended, we are laid asleep

In body, and become a living soul;
While with an eye made quiet by the power
    of harmony, and deep power of joy,
We see into the life of all things.[13]

The thing happened one summer afternoon, on the school cricket field, while I was sitting on the grass, waiting my turn to bat. I was thinking about nothing in particular, merely enjoying the pleasures of midsummer idleness. Suddenly, and without warning, something invisible seemed to be drawn across the sky, transforming the world about me into a kind of tent of concentrated and enhanced significance. What had been merely an outside became an inside. The objective was somehow transformed into a completely subjective fact, which was experienced as mine, but on a level where the word had no meaning – for 'I' was no longer the familiar ego. Nothing more can be said about the experience, it brought no accession of knowledge about anything except, very obscurely, the knower and his way of knowing. After a few minutes there was a 'return to normalcy'. The event made a deep impression on me at the time; but, because it did not fit into any of the thought patterns – religious, philosophical, scientific – with which, as a boy of fifteen, I was familiar, it came to seem more and more anomalous, more and more irrelevant to 'real life', and was finally forgotten.[14]

It is these observable and measurable changes that have allowed for the introduction of meditation as a therapy into several orthodox medical centres. Meditation can be defined as a state of 'relaxed non-aroused physiological functioning' and the changes that have been identified with this state include:

1 Slowing of the pulse
2 Lowering of blood pressure
3 Reduction in breathing rate
4 Increase in blood flow to fingers and toes
5 Changes in oxygen and CO_2 concentrations in the blood
6 Reduction in lactate
7 Alterations in brainwave pattern: (a) increase in alpha brainwave activity (b) synchronisation of brainwaves (left and right hemispheres)

Some of these can be observed during the practice of meditation. Regular practice produces a 'carry-over' effect which has proved effective in the management of several clinical disorders, including migraine, high blood pressure, sleep disturbance, pain relief, anxiety and other stress-related disorders.[15] Far more commonly, however, is the use of meditation as a spiritual exercise and a technique for 'transforming one's consciousness'.

More recent developments have been to explore the link between mental states, the immune system and chronic disorders from arthritis to cancer.[16] Self-help interventions, including relaxation techniques, meditation and visual imagery form part of the therapeutic packages that are associated with 'new-age' therapies. The therapists involved in these interventions are clear that spiritual transformation and personal salvation form an integral part of the expected outcome.

> Through this system a person is able to make contact with his Soul or Divine energies, literally rejuvenating his whole being. In this expanded state of awareness he is easily able to release deep-seated blockages. Not only from this life, early childhood traumas etc., but also from other incarnations. This therapy also helps most physical-emotional-mental-psychic, and sexual conditions.[17]

It is these all-encompassing claims that have led some critics to warn against the returning to an era of religious superstition and the acceptance of a spiritual cause to health and disease. Let us not forget Hippocrates' admonition that 'too many use the divine as a screen for their inability to offer any assistance.'

It is, nevertheless, a fact that the process of mental imagery which is an accepted and legitimate focus of enquiry in cancer treatment is described in detail in the *Spiritual Exercises of Ignatius Loyola* published several centuries before. Whole-person medicine, with its emphasis on integrating body, mind and spirit has emerged in the latter part of the twentieth century as a health-care movement which challenges the bio-medical model of man that has held sway since the time of Descartes and Newton. Its emergence parallels the importance placed on 'man's relationship with himself' that forms an integral part of the Green movement. The wish to 'obey the laws of nature' and 'promises to achieve a higher reason' are pursued by 'Greens' and 'patients' alike through a process of spiritual practice which has been linked with the art of healing that transcends both centuries and cultures.

14

Opting In and Opting Out

The consumer movement is second only to the concern for the environment as a principle feature of the greening process. In health care this has manifested itself in the growth of 'self-care' and self-help groups on the one hand and the increased interest in alternative medicine on the other. Both these developments are not by any means new and, again, it is helpful to place them within an historical context.

At any one time, in most cultures, it is possible to discern three distinct systems of health care operating. *Self-care* involves those steps an individual may take himself regarding his own health care; *Folk-care* involves the use of lay-volunteers and/or those health care practitioners who operate outside the orthodoxy of that particular culture, e.g. alternative or fringe practitioners in the West; and *Professional-care* refers to the established and accepted state system of health care – in the UK this refers to the profession of medicine, nursing, dentistry, midwifery and other allied professions.

Self-care has always formed a major function in the health care of the nation, but until recently has been largely neglected as a serious area for medical research. As has been stated by Fry, 'Without self-care any system of health care would be swamped'.[1] The definition of what constitutes self-care varies, but it can and does involve the following activities – self-diagnosis, self-medication, disease prevention and health maintenance. The extent to which these activities are undertaken has only been realised in the last twenty years and the recognition of the part they play in the total health care of the nation has made academics from all disciplines begin to take notice of the potential that lies within many of these approaches. The impetus towards self-care has received increased emphasis in the last two decades as a result of a number of different factors operating in society, some of which have been referred to earlier. These factors include (a) the loss of prestige enjoyed by the medical profession, (b) the rise of consumerism and the empowerment of the patient, (c) the increase in knowledge and self-education regarding health-care practices, and finally but not least is (d) the erosion of adequate health-care facilities. The provision of professional health-care services for all is a very recent phenomenon even within Western culture. Although 'Folk Medicine' has largely become extinct in England we can still see traces of its influence in the use of the copper bracelet for rheumatism or charms for psoriasis, and it has to be remembered that 80 per cent of the population in Third World countries have no immediate access to professional care, so that self-care and folk-care are their only options.

In the UK, several surveys suggest that self-treatment occurs on average in three out of four episodes of illness.[2] A proportion of people will do nothing, but the majority will take some form of medication. A study in a London estate estimated that, within a four-week period, one in four residents had taken some form of medicine prescribed by their doctor but over two-thirds had taken some form of medication usually bought from a chemist.[3] Other surveys support these findings and suggest that self-prescribed medicines are taken twice as often as those prescribed by doctors. Drugs obtained over the counter (OTC), account for about one third of the total drug bill, and this figure has not altered even with the advent of the National Health Service. Some of the most widely used medications are shown in Figure 15.[4] Surveys conducted amongst GPs suggest that they consider that up to 25 per cent of patients seeking their help could have managed with self-care only, and that a further 18 per cent could usefully have supplemented self-care to the treatment suggested by the doctor.[5] The reasons usually given for not seeking professional advice include the complaint that either it was 'not serious enough' or 'I did not wish to bother the doctor'. It is interesting to note that there are discrepancies between doctors' and patients' views as to whether self-treatment is appropriate or not. However, an attempt by doctors to produce a book offering advice on 'self-treatment' had to be abandoned, as there was no consensus amongst the doctors as to what ailments should be self-treated and which treatment should be recommended.[6] This may reflect the difference between professional medical treatment, which by and large believes there is *one* form of treatment for each condition,

Figure 15 Self-medication drugs consumed in any day (percentage of population)

The groups of OTC drugs most widely consumed are analgesics, vitamins and cough medicines

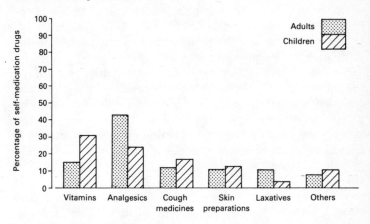

Source: After Kohn and White, (1976).

and lay-beliefs, which will draw on a wide variety of 'folk remedies', 'grandmother's favourites' and 'old wives' tales'.

The variety of remedies used to treat colds has included anything from egg-white, honey, lemon, linseed oil, mint, to stout, whisky and brandy. Clearly an individual could find one item within such a wide list that would meet his need. The antipathy towards 'self-medication' that is to be found amongst professional health-care workers is often stated as relating to the possibility of 'missing the diagnosis' or 'dangerous and harmful treatment'. It is not possible to obtain accurate figures concerning how often self-treatment has delayed adequate professional help, and each doctor will have his own favourite story regarding a headache that turned out to be a brain tumour, or a cough that was not taken sufficiently seriously and was a symptom of pneumonia or lung cancer. Some retrospective studies suggest that only 5 per cent of self-treatment undertaken by patients are thought to be potentially harmful.[7] It is important to place this figure against the known hazards of medical treatment and it is partly because of the higher rate of side-effects and iatrogenic disease that there is an increasing interest in 'folk remedies', which are perceived to be less dangerous than those prescribed by doctors.

The demystification of the medical profession and the general increase in 'anti-technology' and anti-authoritarian attitudes associated with the Green movement will ensure that self-treatment and self-medication will almost certainly increase in the next two decades. The resistance and suspicion towards self-treatment observed amongst health-care professionals need to be viewed not only against the genuine concern over safety issues but in relation to the power-relationship that is being challenged. Self-diagnosis and self-treatment are not activities that are pursued alone. A person's perception of their own symptoms will vary considerably and the level of education and sophistication regarding the significance of symptoms will also vary. Class and cultural factors may have an important bearing on how the patient responds to a set of symptoms, e.g. pinto is a skin disease so prevalent amongst some South American tribes that individuals who do not have this condition consider themselves to be ill. Early morning vomiting, as a sign of pregnancy, is considered at times normal, acceptable and often sought for in Western countries, whilst in certain cultures it is never reported. A survey of women revealed a great difference in the way they felt about their periods. Asked to keep a calendar of symptoms over an eight-week time-scale, 100 per cent of social class I and II women mentioned the onset of periods and symptoms associated with them, whereas 78 per cent of social class IV and V made no mention of periods. When asked why, their answers were invariably that, for them, periods were part of what 'being a woman' was about and not therefore a symptom.[8]

Other factors that may influence our choice regarding self-treatment will be determined by the duration of the symptom and need for legitimisation, e.g., sick certificate and/or the nature of our family and social structure. A study of patients attending a GPs surgery identified that over 85 per cent had sought advice or help from one other person before going to the doctor and 3.5 per cent had had advice from over five different sources. These included friends, spouses, magazines, pharmacists and books. It was considered that the advice given by this wise variety of agencies was sound and appropriate in 75–95 per cent of instances.[9] Thus self-treatment and self-diagnosis are supported by a wide circle of 'lay' or 'voluntary' helpers and these 'unofficial' health-care advisers are found in even greater numbers when one observes the areas of disease prevention and health maintenance.

Disease prevention has been defined as 'specific behaviours or activities which are intended to prevent either the experience or the spread of specific disease'. A good example might be the fluoridation of water as a method of combating dental decay or the wearing of seat-belts to diminish the risk of severe injury. A more extreme form of disease prevention would be the avoidance of car driving altogether as a way of avoiding the risk of road accidents, but clearly this would impose limitations that would be considered unacceptable. Disease prevention is mostly undertaken by health-care personnel, and will include immunisation against measles or tetanus, as well as the screening for high-blood pressure, cervical and breast cancer. The public's perception of these preventive programmes is largely influenced by the level of professional involvement, although some strange anomalies may be observed. If there is universal professional agreement that a preventive measure is helpful, e.g. immunisation or fluoridation, then opposition to that procedure will develop amongst lay groups, either because there is a stated concern over the safety of the intervention or because it is claimed that freedom of choice is being infringed. Similarly, if the medical profession is uncertain as to the value of a particular screening procedure, e.g. cervical smears and breast mammography for the early detection of cancer, there will be a demand from the public which will influence politicians to ensure that such screening procedures are made widely available. Issues of power and control are to be found in almost all areas of health care.

Probably the most important development in disease prevention has been a truly lay activity – the emergence of the self-help group. Over 500 such groups now exist and range from the best known, Alcoholics Anonymous, to the Ileostomy Association. The range and types of groups vary enormously and range from multi-million pound organisations to small informal meetings in someone's front room. Such groups are of two sorts: those which offer a direct service to their client group, either through specific aids, mutual support or direct advice and counselling, and those that fund-raise, mount professional propaganda campaigns and essentially support the 'official' professional health-care model, e.g., Cancer Research Council or National Association for Mental Health. Although both these groupings may serve very different functions, both are the result of the common disadvantage felt by their members.

The self-help movement has demonstrated to the (caring) agencies the therapeutic potency of the process whereby people with similar stigma find each other, strengthen each other through mutual consciousness-raising and support, and express anger about and reject the prevailing modes of professional and societal response to their condition.[10]

The emergence of such groups is a new development in health care, unlike self-treatment which has always been present. As a social phenomenon it is assumed that they have arisen in Western industrialised society as a result of the inadequacies of the health-care services. These inadequacies are indeed present but may be more related to quality than quantity. The mode of health care largely practised in the West is focused on the individual consultation, whether it be the doctor's consulting room, the social worker's private office or the health visitor giving advice to a mother in her own home. The emergence of the self-help group may be a reflection of the need for a communal or group experience similar to the healing ceremonies found in more 'primitive' cultures. Having an illness gives a patient a legitimate 'label' for joining such a group and receiving the supports and benefits that belonging to a group allow. For many, the pursuit of health-maintenance programmes serves a similar function. The enormous increase in yoga classes, keep-fit and jogging, relaxation and meditation groups is an expression of the importance that 'health' and quality of life now play in our national life. They also allow for a connection to be made with other human beings in what is experienced as an increasingly fragmented world.

Thus one of the major influences of the Green movement in medicine is its emphasis on health and health-promoting activities.

What is health?

It seems that even more problematic than defining what constitutes a disease is what constitutes *health*. In *The Short Reign of Pippin IV*, John Steinbeck wrote: 'Pippin was healthy in so far as he knew – by that I mean his health was so good he was not aware he had it.' It does seem that 'healthiness' is more than just 'the absence of disease'. The World Health Organisation arrived at a definition in 1946 which attempted to avoid the link between health and disease. Health is the 'state of complete physical, mental and social well being'. This seems a high ideal and very few people would consider themselves healthy using that definition. Indeed a prominent physician's comment on the WHO definition was that he had only known this state in people who are manic or about to have a heart attack! Could we define health by how long we live, or how happy we are or by how many times we have visited our doctor?

How do ordinary people describe health? These are some definitions taken from a French study:

> My body functions like a well-oiled machine without having to be looked after – and there's also having sparkling eyes, a good colour, feeling at ease when you meet friends and not being on edge.

> I feel strong, able to make an effort, able to keep awake, on top, not tired, not aware of my weakness.

Another Frenchman, describing how he feels when he is healthy, says

> It's able to act so as to do what you want to do, live how you want to live.[11]

It seems that 'healthiness' can, at times, be equated to 'robustness' or 'hardiness' – how much one *can do* and how one copes with the stresses of daily living. On the other hand, health can also be equated to *how one feels*, one's mental attitude and *state of contentment*. To define health, it is necessary to know in what context and what culture the person is living. A more accurate concept may be arrived at if the phrase *comparative health* is used. This suggests that standards of 'healthiness' vary from country to country. Yet another concept is that of *acceptable health*. Such a definition has been provided by Williamson, who writes:

> Acceptable health is a state of perceived well-being whether or not disease or disability is present, provided that the latter does not interfere either with the sufferer's normal life or with that of people whom he or she may affect through community living.[12]

This interest in health and healthy activities is partly the result of the social and economic changes of Western countries that have occurred within the last fifty years. These changes have brought with them their own particular form of diseases. No longer are we having to deal with the problem of infection and malnutrition, but with the chronic conditions of heart disease, arthritis and cancer. Many of these diseases are multifactorial in origin and do not lend themselves to the 'magic bullet' approach to treatment. Some of the factors involved relate to life-style, patterns of exercise and relaxation, diet and dietary imbalances as opposed to malnutrition and bacterial infection. In addition, we have witnessed an epidemic of disorder of mood and desire, so that, increasingly, the role of the health-care practitioner has had to involve health education and behavioural modification. The response from the professional health-care practitioners has been slow and there has been a dramatic increase in the involvement of what can be labelled as the 'popular health movement'. The emphasis on life-style changes is not new and Hippocrates himself was aware of its limitation when he wrote:

> When a carpenter is ill he asks the physician for a rough and ready cure, an emetic or a purge or cautery or the knife, these are his remedies. And if someone prescribes for him a course of dietetics (diet) and exercise and that he must swathe and swaddle his head, and all that sort of thing, he replies at once that he has not time to be ill and that he sees no good of a life spent in nursing his disease to the neglect of his customary employment.

It is clear that Hippocrates felt that health maintenance programmes and life-style advice were only for the affluent, and the modern explosion of interest in these areas seems to support his original observation.

Sylvester Graham, a Pennsylvanian temperance lecturer in the early part of the nineteenth century, founded a movement (Grahamism), the basis of which was the advocacy of vegetarianism, bathing, fresh air, sunlight, dress reform, sex hygiene and abstention from drink.[13] *The Graham Journal*, or *The Health Journal Advocate*, published during his lifetime, could be viewed as the precursor of the myriad of similar publications that can be found in any newsagent's store today. Other journals and societies followed – *The Ladies Physiological Reform Society*, *The Physiology of Marriage* being two typical titles. The movement was so strong that the laws against quackery, 'the irregular practice of medicine', were revoked. In England, similar movements linked to evangelical and social movements developed and in 1828 *The Constitution of Man* was published, which was a treatise on phrenology and its link to health. The movements were often linked to women's rights and, during the early part of the twentieth century, books on marriage, contraception, and natural childbirth began to appear, partly as medical books but partly as socio-political treatises. The era of scientific medicine, with the advances in surgery, pharmacology and anaesthesia, threatened to overwhelm the popular health movement and make its message redundant, for like Hippocrates' carpenter, most people would prefer to take the magic bullet rather than worry about their food, exercise patterns or attitudes. The modern resurgence of this popular movement occurred in the Sixties and, as on previous occasions, it was linked to feminist and political issues. *Our Bodies, Ourselves*[14] was an immediate bestseller and, like Graham's book in the 1820s, heralded a series of similar books, magazines, periodicals, health clubs, jogging groups.

The importance of food in the maintenance of health has had an impact on the health-food industry where now almost every major supermarket has a health-food counter whereas, previously, the purchase of such items was possible only at specialised food stores. Both the popular health movement and the health-food industry have become permanent features in our national life and together with the growth and interest in alternative and complementary therapies form part of the move away from traditional medical-orientated and disease-based models of health-care practice.

Opting out – the alternative health movement

There is little doubt that the most obvious example of the 'greening process' in medicine is the interest and exponential growth of the alternative health movement. The term 'alternative medicine' is not easy to define as it covers a 'pot-pourri' of activities, some requiring rigorous training akin to medicine, others faltering on the edge of deceit and charlatanism. The term is usually defined as 'including all those therapies and approaches to healing that are not covered by the traditional undergraduate curriculum'.[15] The word complementary is used by some as a way of avoiding the confrontation with traditional medicine. The term 'holistic' has been taken over by the alternative movement to the extent that it has lost any of its original meaning. Other epithets include Natural Medicine or Green Medicine, which immediately give it the link with the Green movement. Indeed books on Green issues refer to the growth of alternative medicine as the medicine of the Green movement. Such a simplistic linking makes it difficult at times to explore and evaluate the claims made by alternative practitioners, and polarised positions on both sides of the argument are easily observed. The following model may help to separate out the myriad of activities that shelter under the umbrella of alternative medicine.[16]

Group 1: Complete systems of healing   These are systems of healing which have a theoretical base as to the causation of disease. They have a diagnostic, investigative and therapeutic understanding which share some similarities with orthodox medicine. Some of these systems have been around for many thousands of years, others are relatively new. The major categories that are found in the UK to any great degree are:

1 Acupuncture or traditional Chinese medicine
2 Herbal medicine
3 Osteopathy
4 Chiropractic
5 Homoeopathy

Most of these systems of healing have an educational framework, publish ethical guidelines and attempt to regulate their practitioners in the same way as the General Medical Council might regulate doctors. They consider themselves, by and large, to be competent enough to deal with most of the problems that come their way, although the more sensible ones tend to suggest that most acute and life-threatening problems are better dealt with by orthodox medicine. Other systems of healing not included in this list are Naturopathy or Ayurvedic medicine – the traditional healing model in India.

Group 2: Diagnostic methods   These are ways of determining the presence or absence of disease using methods not normally linked with traditional medicine, e.g.

1 Kinesiology – as a test for allergies
2 Iridology – as a test for hidden disease

3 Hair analysis – as a test for nutritional defects
4 Aura diagnosis – as a test for levels of well-being.

There are many such methods, some not requiring the presence of the patient, such as intuitive diagnosis; some that claim to
be 'scientific' and use many splendid-looking machines; others
that claim to call on powers 'unknown to science'. Anecdotal
evidence is easy to find, but any substantial body of evidence is
absent. Indeed, iridology as a method of diagnosis has been
discredited in a reputable trial.

Group 3: Therapeutic modalities   These treatments again are
not found in traditional medicine, and the list is endless. Most
practitioners of these therapies do not claim any diagnostic skill
but they do claim that their treatments can and do work. It is
probably within this group that the term complementary is most
suitable. The treatments 'complement' or 'supplement' what is
already on offer. This group includes:

1 Massage – or therapeutic touch
2 Reflexology
3 Aromatherapy
4 Spiritual healing
5 Hydrotherapy

Group 4: Self-help measures   This group includes the package of
self-help measures where patients are encouraged to undertake
certain practices and exercises that will either diminish their
symptoms, improve their health or maintain their well-being.
These self-help measures include:

1 Breathing and relaxation techniques
2 Meditation
3 Visualisation
4 Yoga and other exercise routines
5 Fasting or dieting, etc.

The alternative movement received a major boost in 1983 when
HRH The Prince of Wales gave his valedictory address as President of the BMA. The Royal Family has always had an interest and
involvement with homoeopathy and osteopathy and when the
Prince said, 'Human nature is such that we are frequently prevented from seeing that what is taken for today's unorthodoxy is

probably tomorrow's convention,' many people understood his reference to be directed towards these therapies. He referred to 'those ancient, unconscious forces, lying beneath the surface which still help to shape the psychological attitudes of modern man' and indicated his understanding of the current criticisms of modern medicine – 'The whole imposing edifice of modern medicine, for all its breathtaking success is like the celebrated Tower of Pisa – slightly off-balance.' His speech attracted wide publicity and acted as the required catalyst for a number of important, clinical, educational, organisational and political changes.

A number of questionnaire surveys revealed an interest amongst doctors which was unrecognised. Reilly (1983) found a positive attitude in 86 of 100 general practitioner trainees towards alternative medicine.[17] Wharton and Lewith (1986), in their survey of 200 general practitioners in the Avon District, found that 38 per cent had received some additional training in some of these activities, and 76 per cent had referred patients to colleagues practising some form of alternative or complementary medicine.[18] The last major survey in the UK in 1982 identified a total of 30,000 practitioners of one sort or another.[19] Subsequent developments have suggested a growth of 10 per cent a year which would make the figure nearer 50,000. However, in what is considered the mainstream of alternative medicine (Group 1), there are no more than 3,000–4,000. If the figure of 20,000 spiritual healers is correct, it suggests that most of the public seeks help from alternative practitioners because scientific rational medicine does not address itself to problems of the spirit. Surveys as to why patients seek alternative medicine do not always provide a coherent set of answers. The consumer magazine Which?, in its survey of almost 2,000 readers, found that one in seven had visited a complementary/alternative practitioner in the previous year, 82 per cent claiming to have improved or been cured, 81 per cent of patients identified dissatisfaction due to poor symptom relief as the main reason for seeking help, 71 per cent sought help for joint or pain problems, 15 per cent sought help for psychological problems.[20] A survey in the Netherlands (Table 15) showed that one in five people have consulted a complementary practitioner.[21]

A more recent survey in the UK carried out by MORI in 1989 shows that 74 per cent of the sample surveyed (1,826 adults) would

Table 14 Numbers of complementary therapists in the UK (1981/2)

Therapy	Medically qualified	In professionl association	Not in professional association	Total
Acupuncture	160	548	250	958
Alexander (Teachers)	5	170	50	225
Chiropractic	1	156	200	357
Hakims, Chinese Doctors	0	40	40	80
Healing	20	6,300	13,000	19,320
Herbalism	10	228	200	438
Homoeopathy	425	41	230	696
Hypnotherapy	1,000	507	170	1,677
Massage/ manipulation	350	1,000	1,500	2,850
Misc. Physical Therapies	0	300	800	1,100
Music/Art/Drama Therapy	0	815	90	905
Naturopathy	5	204	200	409
Osteopathy	212	777	150	1,139
Radionics	21	98	100	219
Total	2,209	11,184	16,980	30,373

Notes: 1 'Misc. Physical Therapies' includes reflexology, rolfing, metamorphic therapy, polarity therapy and applied kinesiology. Since there are no proper professional bodies with registers in these therapies, and they are taught to the public, the number given in column 2 is an estimate of the number of instructors plus full-time practitioners. The number in column 3 is an estimate of the part-time and occasional practitioners. All estimates are derived from the organisations themselves.

2 Art, music and drama therapies are included as they are arguably alternatives to conventional rehabilitation and are based more on anthroposophical than medical principles.

3 Massage/manipulation excludes beauty therapists.

4 Certain other therapies such as colour, aroma, sound therapies are not specifically included, but practitioners have been incorporated into the estimates in column 3 of naturopathy, homoeopathy and herbalism.

5 'Medically qualified' implies doctors. However, as organisations mostly failed to distinguish between doctors and other health professionals, it is possible that in some cases paramedical and auxiliary medical professionals will also have been included in column 1. Otherwise they would be included in column 2 or 3.

Source: S. Fulder, *The Handbook of Complementary Medicine* (1984).

Table 15 Numbers of people consulting therapists of various disciplines in the Netherlands

Theory	% of sample of 689	% of Dutch adult population
Homoeopathy	37·7	6.9
Healing	35·5	6.5
Naturopathy	18.9	3·4
Herbalism	16.7	3.0
Chiropractic and osteopathy	13.2	2.4
Acupuncture	11.6	2.1
Yoga therapy	6.1	1.1
Anthroposophical medicine	2.9	0.5
Others	3.8	0.7

Notes: 1 689 people out of the 3,782 adult members of the public polled at random had been to see a complementary practitioner.

2 The figures add up to more than 100 per cent as some people have seen more than one kind of practitioner.

Source: S. Fulder *op cit*. (1984)

like to see some forms of alternative medicine introduced into the Health Service. However, 69 per cent had not had any experience of alternative treatments and only 10 per cent had tried either homoeopathy or osteopathy.[22]

As a direct result of The Prince of Wales' intervention, the BMA appointed a Scientific Committee to report on the efficacy of alternative medicine in England. Its precise remit was: 'To consider the feasibility and possible methods of assessing the value of alternative therapies, whether used alone or to complement other treatments.'[23]

The membership of the working party was drawn from within the BMA and surprisingly contained no person familiar with the subject and no general practitioner. The Committee sent out requests to a number of different bodies asking for information. Initially the time given for these bodies to respond was very small (eight weeks) and many of the established groups declined to take part. Over 600 submissions were received and the Committee also heard oral evidence. At the end of 1984, after a number of revisions, it produced its report and conclusions. It would be very easy to dismiss the validity of the report given that it was conducted in such a haphazard way. Equally the lack of any informed member on the Committee made it almost impossible for the group to assess the relative merit of the evidence submitted. Nevertheless the report identified certain factors which they felt were common to a number of alternative therapies and were important to acknowledge. These factors were:

(1) *Time*: alternative practitioners were able to offer patients more time to listen – the complaint that doctors were too busy was heard over and over again.

(2) *Compassion*: as well as being given time, patients felt alternative practitioners were more caring and concerned. They treated the 'whole person' and not the disease.

(3) *Touch*: in many of the alternative therapies, touch is used: e.g., massage, reflexology, acupressure, laying on of hands. This very fundamental method of communicating healing was thought by the BMA to contrast with the technology of modern medicine which got in the way of the doctor and patient.

(4) *Authority and Charisma*: as medicine had become more familiar, it seemed important for patients to seek out practitioners who appeared 'magical'. Many of the alternative therapies with their strange words and unfamiliar practices conveyed the atmosphere of a magical cult which was a very powerful healing force.

As one can see from the above description, the BMA, whilst acknowledging that alternative medicine was growing in popularity, thought it was doing so because modern medicine was failing to give patients something they wanted. The Committee generally felt that the scientific validity of the therapies themselves was almost impossible to demonstrate. Partly this was because the sorts of problems seen by alternative practitioners were episodic (they relapsed and recurred naturally) and were non-life-threatening. They were unable to find clear evidence of a *scientific* kind to prove, for instance, that acupuncture worked in asthma or that homoeopathy was of help in psoriasis. They also felt that to conduct such studies would be difficult and costly. However, they did acknowledge that the weight of descriptive evidence for acupuncture in pain relief and osteopathy and chiropractic in back problems was so great that they accepted that these therapies did indeed have a place in the proper management of these disorders. Similarly they supported hypnotherapy, biofeed-back and some forms of dietary therapy, in a limited set of circumstances.

A further initiative was undertaken by the Royal Society of Medicine, which under the then President, Sir James Watt, hosted a series of 'Colloquia'. A series of dialogues between alternative practitioners and medical practitioners took place which were summarised and eventually published.[24] As a result of these 'Colloquia' and subsequent meetings hosted by HRH The Prince of Wales, some of the suspicion and rancour between the two groups of practitioners diminished and substantive steps were taken to ensure adequate training and evaluation of the more established complementary therapies. Developments in the European Community meant that legislation regarding the acceptance and registration of complementary practitioners has been accelerated by the approaching deadline of 1992. This, together with the consumer interest, has ensured that several of the therapies and therapists involved in alternative medicine will achieve official recognition by the State if not by the orthodox medical profession. Several attempts to integrate both approaches to health care have been made, most notably at the Marylebone Health Centre (see Chapter 15). It will be interesting to observe, as the therapies are absorbed into the State system, whether their appeal to the public will diminish, for there is no doubt that part of the appeal is that the therapies *are* an alternative to the traditional model of health care. If they are integrated within the traditional model, some of that appeal may disappear. A not dissimilar phenomenon is occurring within the Green movement. As their policies and approaches are becoming accepted by the establishment political parties, so the energy and fervour of their supporters have diminished.

15

The Seeds Begin to Sprout

So far we have explored certain developments in medical care that focused on a particular condition and its treatment – the management of the terminally ill or the approach to pregnancy. All these developments have affected the care of patients in a substantial way. Nevertheless, for the majority of patients in the UK, the first contact with medicine is through general practice. This particular discipline of medicine has undergone rapid and fundamental changes in the last thirty years and is about to enter into a further phase of development as a result of the White Paper and the new GP contract. The uniqueness and strength of British medicine comes in part as the direct result of the central place general practice has in the organisational framework of health delivery. Any defect in the discipline will affect the lives of millions. Similarly the improvements that are now occurring have potential widespread benefits. It is because of this unique position that experiments in primary health care that challenge the traditional model of general practice are so important. Three such experiments are outlined below and each has had much to contribute to the 'greening' process in medical care. The first attempted to rethink the delivery of health care in a truly revolutionary way and started with a premise which recognised the importance of health as opposed to disease.

The Peckham Experiment

The pilot phase of this extraordinary experiment began in 1926. By the time it closed, it was attracting over 10,000 visitors a year. Its founders, Dr George Scott Williamson and Dr Innes Pearse, were in great demand as speakers and lecturers all over the world. The hypothesis they set up to test was that 'health is more infectious than disease'. They believed that if they provided an environment where individuals could come and participate in 'healthy activities', during which time they could be provided with 'periodic healthy examination' including information on how to promote their health; their quality of life would improve.[1]

The second major focus for the experiment was that it should be centred on families and not individuals, for they believed that the 'creative' and containing environment for each individual was his family. They felt that even though individual health services were important and helpful in both detecting and treating disease – 'if the individual returns to the same environmental conditions from which the disorder sprung', then either the problem would recur or a further difficulty would manifest itself in time. Included in the term 'environment' was the individual's family and, equally important, the architecture of the building they lived in (see below). Thirdly, both doctors believed that individual responsibility was not only a biological characteristic of the human species but that any system that discouraged this individual responsibility was essentially unhealthy. They therefore attempted to reduce the bureaucracy, committee structure and any semblance of central authority. Thus the only two rules included

1 All members of the family had to join and agree to a periodic health overhaul – the cost of membership initially was one shilling (5p).
2 Use of the centre's equipment and activities were free to all children under five and of school age, but adults had to pay an extra charge for each activity.

The experiment initially began in a small health centre in South London. It operated as a form of 'club' and thirty families came together to organise it. It rapidly outgrew its accommodation and a new purpose-built building – the pioneer health centre – was designed and built in 1935. The building was constructed of concrete and glass, way ahead of its time. The three storeys accommodated the medical, administrative and recreational facilities. The latter included a swimming pool, cafeteria, games room, bar, quiet rooms and library. One of the principles of the design was visibility and much use was made of glass, both for internal and external partitions. The visibility was partly to ensure that members could observe each other participating in activities they themselves may have been unwilling to entertain, e.g., swimming, and partly to allow the medical and research staff to observe the activities without interfering with them unduly. In addition to encouraging 'change initiated by the sight of action', all parts of the building were freely accessible and available to all. This again encouraged intermingling of different groups and different generations. There was maximum use of the different spaces for differing activities and no one place was designed for only one purpose except for the swimming pool. The gymnasium was used for theatre, dance, lectures, as well as sporting activities. Decisions as to the use of these facilities were determined by the members and not the 'authorities'. The building was both an expression of the experiment as well as a laboratory designed for the study of family behaviour. The staff avoided becoming involved in organising, suggesting or promoting any of the recreational activities and limited themselves to responding to direct requests for facts and information from the members.

The health overhauls were arranged at times of mutual convenience and involved individual and family interviews. Doctors undertook both physical and laboratory checks on all members and then discussed these openly with all members of the family. Treatment and advice were not given or focused on, and referral to other doctors and hospitals was suggested if any specific disease was discovered. The medical directors of the centre felt that the most likely 'points of change' within both an individual or family were when life transitions occurred, e.g., marriage, birth, going to school, adolescence, retirement, and wherever possible, members were encouraged to have an 'overhaul' at these critical points. It is important to understand that these 'overhauls' were focused on encouraging health and not on discovering disease.

Thus while medical overhaul culminates in advice and treatment given in respect of action to be taken by the patient, health overhaul culminates in producing information for the subject to use at his own discretion. In the first the examiner retains his traditional role as doctor, responsible for determining the procedure of the patient seeking advice. In the second he is acting like the family's bank manager informing his client as to 'where he stands and what he can stretch to'. These are the words in which members of the centre often explained to visitors what the centre 'doctors do'.[2]

Dr Scott Williamson and Dr Pearse published their first findings in 1938 and 1943. They had found, at the time of joining as members, that only 9 per cent of individuals were found to have 'nothing wrong'. Ninety-one per cent were shown to have some treatable condition ranging from minor deformities, e.g., carious teeth, to cancers. These figures were obtained before the Second World War and before the National Health Service. It was assumed that with the introduction of free care and free access that the level of undisclosed and undiscovered diseases would fall. Figures obtained more recently suggest that this is not so, and that the NHS has not improved the health and well-being of the population to the degree that had been hoped. The belief that underpinned the Pioneer Health Centre was that by providing regular information to individuals and families about their state of health and providing a social environment where engaging in health activities was visibly encouraged, then the path to recovery and increasing health was facilitated. At the height of its functioning, there were between 500 and 1,000 people every night at the centre and the crucial lesson of responsibility in health seems to have been learned early by the directors.

> Our failures during the first eighteen months work taught us something very significant. Individuals from infants to old people resent or fail to show any interest in anything initially presented to them through discipline, regulation or instruction. We now proceed by merely providing an environment rich in instrument for action, that is, giving a chance to do things. Slowly but surely these chances are seized upon and used as opportunities for development of inherent capacity. The instruments of action have one common characteristic – they must speak for themselves.[3]

It was hoped that, with the onset of the NHS, some of the principles embodied by the Peckham Experiment would be incorporated within the planning of the new health centres due to be built. Neither the importance of design of building nor the participatory nature of the experiment and, more importantly, the focus on health was seen as important. The health centres built within the NHS were managed and organised by doctors – the service offered was a reactive disease-based model and the preventive and promotional focus was minimised. With the death of the pioneers of the Peckham Experiment, much of the impetus for their method of work was lost and attempts to keep the model alive have proved difficult and problematic. The reasons for this are complex and are not solely due to the resistance of the medical profession or intransigence of the health authorities. A disease-based service is sought by the majority of the public, and to offer a health-based service, without offering treatment for the diseases uncovered, does limit the practicality of the model. In addition, although the Peckham Experiment was based on an understanding of human systems, i.e. the individual functioning within a family, and the families functioning within the community, it failed to recognise that the experiment itself was part of a larger system which involved 'official' health-care administrators and politicians. It thus neglected to develop its links with the 'external systems' required to ensure its survival. Any 'centre of excellence' that wishes to survive and see its influence develop beyond its own boundaries needs to keep its own boundaries open to the external realities that exist in the society it finds itself in. A 'centre' that remains 'closed' to these realities will find itself starved of resources eventually. Any new model of health care must take into account the social, economic and political framework within which it has to operate. Earlier in this book I described the 'languages' now required to ensure the growth of any new venture of this kind. The Peckham pioneers avoided the language of the politician and the health economist and, probably more critically, failed to grasp the need to talk in the language of disease and illness.

A further experiment in delivering primary health care which tries to incorporate some of the ideas initiated at the Pioneer Health Centre is the one being undertaken in the converted crypt of a church at Marylebone.

The Marylebone Health Centre

The original work that developed into the innovative General Practice Unit at Marylebone began in 1984 with a pilot research project on self-care that took place at Lisson Grove Health Centre in Paddington.[4] This project evaluated the outcome of introducing a series of self-care classes (breathing and relaxation, exercise, meditation) into a project; the Wates Foundation made a further five-year grant to develop the work. This required moving the clinical and research unit out of its original base at Lisson Grove to a new purpose-built practice. At about the same time, the Reverend Christopher Hamel-Cooke, rector of St Marylebone

Parish Church, had the inspired wish to convert the crypt of the church into a 'healing centre'. He had long felt the need to build new bridges between religion and medicine and felt the vast warren of unused space could be utilised to bridge the gap between body and soul. The concept behind the Reverend Hamel-Cooke's idea was supported by highly influential church and medical personalities. When I met the rector, it became clear within an hour of our exchange that our two 'visions' were sufficiently compatible to ensure that the difficulties and hurdles were overcome without too many problems. The original objective of the research project funded by Wates was

> to explore and evaluate ways in which primary health care can be delivered to an inner city area in addition to the General Practice component. The 'new' approaches to include an holistic component comprising an educational self-help model with a complementary medical model.

Like the Peckham Experiment, we were very concerned to ensure that the design and structure of the conversion reflected the 'containment and bringing together' that was part of our shared philosophy. The two architects, Nicki and John Braithwaite, were particularly well-chosen having worked on the Snape Concert Hall and the conversion of Southwark's Holy Trinity Church. Both architects sought to retain as much of the existing vaulted crypt structure. The former vaults lent themselves well to small counselling rooms and the design has attempted to offer a supportive sense of being together.

The crypt had been the final resting place for 850 Victorian parishioners and when permission was granted for the bodies to be removed to Brookwood Cemetery, it could literally be said that the dead had given way to the living. When the centre was opened by HRH The Prince of Wales in July 1987, it housed four separate units – the pastoral centre, the NHS general practice, with its research unit, a music therapy unit, and the most advanced of 'high-tech' units, a magnetic resonance imaging centre, able to provide the most detailed body scans then available. The general practice is the core of the centre, providing primary health care, much like any other general practice. It has two general practitioners and the usual complement of staff found in most modern practices (nurses, counsellors, health visitors, midwives etc). Local patients register with the practice in the normal way, and it became clear fairly quickly that the practice population included a much higher proportion of the underprivileged and disadvantaged groups than normally found. Although situated in a relatively privileged part of London, the practice profile is atypical in that it contains both the wealthy middle-class professional and the poor, the unemployed, the homeless and the ethnic minorities. The research and audit unit linked to the practice provides a highly developed computer facility which supports all elements of the work.

We need to be constantly testing out what we are doing – for example, conducting research on how complementary therapies work within general practice and comparing their use in treating specific conditions.[5]

It is the complementary therapy unit which has attracted much of the publicity at Marylebone. The latter can draw on the skills of an osteopath, homoeopath, traditional Chinese practitioner, massage therapist, stress counsellor and herbalist. After an initial consultation with a GP, patients may be referred to one of the complementary practitioners. In addition, a special multi-disciplinary clinic is held weekly, where practitioners from different disciplines will both see and discuss patients together. These patients with complex and intractable problems may have referred themselves or been referred by individual practitioners.

At my first visit the practice nurse discovered that I was suffering from hypertension and this was duly reported to the doctor. After a series of questions concerning my life-style, I was asked if instead of being prescribed powerful drugs, I would be prepared to embark on a programme of relaxation and diaphragmatic breathing exercises.

Now some months later, I can honestly say with sincerity and some amazement, that the benefits have transformed my life in ways which I would not have thought possible.[6]

The 'patients' are encouraged and invited to participate in a range of activities which are intended to ensure an active participation in the running of the health centre. A practice register of 'befrienders' together with a list of services that can be offered (baby-sitting, help with transport, translating and legal work, etc) is available to all patients and special groups (parents and children, single-parents, the homeless and the elderly) have been organised by the 'users committee' which writes and produces the three-monthly newsletter. The aims of this outreach and community programme are not only to bring people into groups at the centre but to put patients and users in touch with community activities outside: a community network is thus created. 'One of the most important things to me in Marylebone Health Centre is that patients have a say in what happens in their health centre.'[7]

The centre organises a comprehensive educational programme of courses that fall into two areas – self-help groups for patients with specific problems (e.g., hypertension, asthma, cancer), and activities promoting positive mental, physical and social health, (e.g., yoga classes, movement to music, relaxation and meditation). The aim of the programme is to encourage and enable patients to take control of their own health and well-being. A users group has been established to provide ideas and feedback on activities. 'The most important thing for me is to improve a sense of well-being in patients, informing and encouraging them but also sharing the power of knowledge.'[8]

To enable such a complex and comprehensive range of activities to take place within and alongside a busy NHS general practice has required a commitment on the part of the staff both at a personal and professional level. Regular meetings, together with twice-yearly residential 'retreats', form part of an active staff development programme.

I think I was first attracted to work here because I believed in change from within – both for myself and for the kind of health care system I wanted to be part of.[9]

Marylebone Health Centre is a normal NHS centre and it uses a 'whole person' approach to health care. It is not only concerned about the health of its patients but also cares about the well-being of its staff.[10]

These supportive comments must be viewed in part as the result of the initial enthusiasm that the formation of a new unit with plentiful resources is bound to create. The detailed evaluative work required to support some of the claims has yet to be completed. From some of the initial audits on prescribing rates, admission and referrals to hospitals, it appears that the 'Marylebone Model' of delivering primary health care may well result in substantial alteration in the use of the traditional end-point of most general practice consultation, i.e., a prescription and/or referral to hospital.

The financial savings on the reduction in prescribing is shown to be consistent, and will go a long way to meet the cost of the additional staff required to run the comprehensive services offered.

The practical implementation of the Marylebone Model illustrates some of the essential features of the 'greening process'. The importance of the context or the environment is illustrated by the very detailed practice and community profile that is available. The knowledge allows for the identification of the 'ecology' of Marylebone and encourages the appropriate husbanding of resources. It allows for connections to be made between different parts of the system, i.e. linking 'patients' with unmet needs, e.g. transport, with patients willing to provide them.

The involvement of the 'patients', 'clients', 'users' in both administrative, organisational and decision-making allows for both horizontal and vertical hierarchies to complement each other. This move towards 'consumerism' within the daily practice of health care is slow and requires fundamental changes in behaviour on the part of all concerned.

The availability of 'alternative therapies' so often linked with Green medicine does make it possible to avoid the use of drugs and increases the human element in the interchange between client and practitioner. The two most often used alternative therapies are massage and counselling (touch and talk). Finally that the experiment is taking place within a church is a reminder of the importance of 'spirituality' in health care. The search for 'wholeness' necessitates a search that can only take place within the depths of our being, however we choose to call this place. This 'inner journey' is available to patients if they wish to pursue it through the various meditational meetings, quiet times, healing services and pastoral counselling available.

The Marylebone experiment like the Peckham experiment has a number of audiences, each with different needs and requirements and each speaking a different language. The success or failure of the Marylebone experiment will, in part, depend on how able we are to listen to the different audiences and how able we are to converse in their language, and not privilege our own particular position. The audiences include, first, *the patients* (to whom the Marylebone Health Centre is the source of their medical care). Is

Peckham Experiment	Marylebone Model	Glyncorrwg Community Practice
1 Our concept (is) that health is a mutual synthesis of organism and environment.	1 There is an interconnectness between human beings and their environment.	1 We must accept the full implications of both groups and individuals practising an open style of medicine.
2 In this new field there was as yet no existing knowledge of well-defined entities, relationships, dynamics and regularities which the bionomist might encounter.	2 Tolerating un-certainty, taking risks and making mistakes are part of the stepping stones in the search for wholeness.	2 We need to admit to ourselves, our colleagues and our patients what we don't yet know and what we haven't yet done.
3 Approaching conventionally as a scientist, how then is he to fulfil the technological requirements of assessment – how is he to measure his material?	3 Research studies should pay due cognisance to the moral, ethical and financial consequences of their outcome. This does not mean that we discard 'science', rather that we respond imaginatively and creatively as scientists to discover the construction of health and disease as a social process.	3 We must learn to apply scientific principles imaginatively to the health care of millions of people as they actually live and work.
4 It is essential to grasp that the processes that sustain and develop an individual's health care other than the processes that underlie	4 Health and disease lie along a continuum and represent the organic-intrinsic state of harmony with the universe.	4 We must learn to deal with measurable, continuously distributed variables in which disease (requiring active remedial inter-

Peckham Experiment	Marylebone Model	Glyncorrwg Community Practice
and govern his disease.		vention) is difficult or even impossible to separate from health (requiring active conservation).
5 Supper is an important time of meeting for all members of the staff. At times these lead to discussions that may run deep.	5 It will not be possible for doctors to address the health problems of the 21st century unless we learn how to share our power, not only amongst our colleagues in the health team but also with our patients.	5 We must accept that effective medical care and even more the effective conservation of health requires an enormous range of skills other than those of doctors, including skills of other medical, nursing and health professionals who have been systematically subordinated to and exploited by us and our predecessors and that our own skills will survive only if they can be shown to be useful.
6 Health of which we were in search, demanded that the family should shoulder the responsibility for its own actions – this was basic to the hypothesis on which the work was conceived.	6 Users of health care services need to be offered knowledge, skills and support to enable them to take an active interest in their health and emotional well-being. They can also share the responsibility for helping to maintain the organisation designed to promote health and community care.	6 We must accept patients as colleagues in a jointly designed and performed production in which they will nearly always have to do most of the work. We must look to a more dependable alliance with the ordinary people we serve.

Marylebone able to respond to the needs of a displaced Bangla-deshi family living in a hotel room at the same time as that of an 'enlightened' journalist seeking acupuncture for her mid-life crisis?

The second audience is the *members of the medical profession* who look on partly in amusement, some with envy, others with scepticism at this experiment. Their language is that of the academic research paper. How effective is massage in treating loneliness? What controls were used for the study on the use of acupuncture in asthma? How selected is the practice population etc? All these questions are valid and need to be answered in the language they are couched in.

The third audience consists of *health-care administrators and politicians* who need to know whether the Marylebone Model is cost-effective and replicable, or another 'atypical centre doing its own thing'. Their questions are addressed in the language of the Nineties – medical audit, consultation rates, prescribing costs, outcome evaluation and patient satisfaction.

The fourth audience includes the *media* – television, press and radio. Their language often will include images of the church, spiritual healing, massage and, of course, the Royal Connection. All this makes good copy and good television. The more serious reporting does also occur but to capture the application of Systems Theory in General Practice in an inner city can be a challenge to even the most creative journalist.

The final audience Marylebone needs to address is *the participants in the experiment itself* – not the patients but the professional practitioners, the receptionists and administrators, the researchers and secretarial staff. How have their needs been met by Marylebone? How nurturing and containing is the environment of Marylebone? How do the conflicts, stresses and power issues get addressed?

It is clear that it would require a most amazing set of circumstances and, indeed, personnel if these questions were to be fully responded to. But by recognising the different systems operating, it may at least be possible to identify the failures and limitations of the model as it develops and expands.

Providing a whole range of services like some health-care supermarket is to parody and devalue the process required to communicate the sense of 'containment' that such experimental units are able to provide. It is interesting to record that the Peckham Experiment arrived at much the same conclusion:

> This raises the question of how to assemble 'wholes' in an experimental context. The mere aggregation of *all* parts does not make a 'whole' – 'All' is a quantitative term which rests on the assembly of a sum total of units. Wholes rests on specific actional relationships not of part to part but of parts to the organisation which the parts constitute.

The Glyncorrwg Community Practice

Unlike the Marylebone Health Centre, the community practice at Glyncorrwg has been functioning for over three decades. The pioneering work undertaken by its senior partner, Dr Julian Tudor-Hart, has been well recorded in the medical literature.[11] The community in Glyncorrwg, a South Wales village, was very closely involved with the mining industry but suffered like many industrial communities by the loss of its main source of employment. In 1966, 92 per cent of men aged 16–64 were gainfully employed but by 1986, this percentage had dropped to 48. A more different community than Marylebone could hardly be envisaged. Yet Dr Tudor-Hart has emphasised the importance of social organisational cohesion on the health of a community and has emphasised the need to foster a new kind of doctor to meet the needs of the next few decades. He draws attention to the importance of the family group and community involvement in helping to sustain the health of individuals, and suggests that doctors need to move away from a reactive, individually based, clinically orientated practice of medicine to one which is proactive, family and community based and which accepts the social, cultural, economic and political factors that influence health and disease. His critique of doctors and governments alike draws on a Marxist view of society and he is highly suspicious of the liberal and humanistic influence on health care, reserving his particular passion and wit for what he sees as their limitation:

> The Liberal critique . . . of scholarly backing, humane intentions, appeal to both left and right intellectual radicals, without embarrassment to either and ability to interpret defeat as victory, is a savage description, but anger is justified, not because these three conclusions are untrue, but because of the

increasingly obvious social and political context in which only these truths have been proclaimed, while others, less convenient to this scoundrel time, have been forgotten. The Liberal Critique has disarmed professional resistance first to revision then to destruction of the post-war social settlement of which the NHS was an important part.[12]

In the final chapter to his book, Tudor-Hart contrasts the requirements he advocates for the 'new kind of doctor' with those usually identified with Sir William Osler – 'the most influential advocate of the professional model – the scientistic medical gentleman'. It is interesting to compare the characteristics of the 'new medicine' as preached and/or practised in the three examples of 'seeds' given so far. What they all seem to have in common is the search for the 'connections' as opposed to 'causes' of health and disease.

The greening process is primarily a search for connection and the exploration of relationships, both animate and inanimate. If the practice of medicine is to pursue these developments, then the work of these three pioneering units will need to be replicated in the context of the lives of the ordinary citizen of this planet, whether in the developed world of the North or the disadvantaged world of the South. The principles underpinning this 'new medicine' can take root only in a cultural environment where the drive for perfection is informed by the pursuit of the ordinary.

References

1 New Gods – Old Worlds

1 Reich, C. *The Greening of America* Penguin 1971
2 Porritt, J. and Winner, D. *The Coming of the Greens* Fontana 1988
3 Capra, F. and Spretnak, C. *Green Politics* E. P. Dutton NY 1984
4 Cousins, N. *Anatomy of an Illness* Norton NY 1979
5 Segal, B. *Love, Medicine and Miracles* Century 1988
6 Le San, L. *You Can Fight for Your Life* Norton NY 1979
7 Vrooman, J. R. *René Descartes* Penguin NY 1970

2 The Origins of Green Ideas

1 Haekel, E. *Last Words on Evolution* Owen, 1906
2 Haekel, E. *The Riddles of the Universe* Watts, 1900
3 Haekel, E. *The Wonders of Life* Watts, 1905
4 *Ibid.*
5 Lovelock, J. *Gaia – A New Look at Life on Earth* OUP 1979
6 *Ibid.*
7 Lovelock, J. *The Ages of Gaia* OUP 1988
8 Weiss, P. *The Science of Life – The Living System* Futura 1973
9 Miller, J. G. *Living Systems* McGraw Hill NY 1978
10 Engel, G. 'The Need for a New Medical Model – A Challenge for Bio-Medicine' *Science 196* 8 April 1977, pp. 129–136
11 Engel, G. 'The Clinical Application of the Biopsychosocial Model *Am. J. Psychiatry 137* 5 May 1980, pp. 535–544
12 Pietroni, P. C. 'The Meaning of Illness' *J. Royal Society of Medicine 80*, 1987 pp. 357–360
13 Smuts, J. *Holism and Evolution*, Macmillan, 1926
14 Koffka, K. *Principles of Gestalt Psychology* Routledge & Kegan Paul 1935

15 Pietroni, P. 'Holistic Medicine – New Map, Old Territory' *Brit.J. of Holistic Medicine* 1, 1984, pp. 3–13

3 The Magic Bullet Begins to Hurt

1 *Congressional Record of the United States* V.XXV. No. 11, 274

2 Boussel, P., Bonneman, H., Bove, F. *History of Pharmacy* Asklepros Press 1982

3 Williamson, J. and Danaher, K. *Self-Care in Health* Croom Helm 1978

4 Withers, C. 'The Folklore of a Small Town' *Transactions of the New York Academy of Science*, Series II 8, 1946 p. 234

5 *The Future for Pharmaceuticals* Office of Health Economics 1983

6 Medawar, C. *The Wrong Kind of Medicine* Hodder & Stoughton 1984

7 Fry, J., Brock, D. and McColl, I. *NHS Data Book* MTP Press 1984

8 *Ibid.*

9 Medawar, C. *op.cit.*

10 Griffin, J. P., Diggle, G. E. *A Survey of Products Licensed in the United Kingdom from 1971–1981* 1981 12(4) *Br.J. Clin. Pharmacol* pp. 453–463

11 Medawar, C. *op.cit.*

12 Maronde, R. F., Lee, P. V., McCarron, M. *et al.* 'A Study of Prescribing Patterns' *Medical Care* 9, 1974 pp. 383–395

13 Parish, P. *Medicines – A Guide for Everybody* 4th Ed. Penguin 1982

14 Inglis, B. 'The Health Services' *Guardian* 24 December 1982

15 Medawar, C. *op.cit.*

16 Illich, I. *Limits to Medicine* Pelican 1977

17 Stimson, G. C., Webb, B. *Going to See the Doctor* Routledge & Kegan Paul 1975

18 Smith, M., Maples, R. E. A. *Prescribing Practice and Drug Usage* Croom Helm 1980

19 'Regional Differences in Medicine Usage in the UK' *Pharmacy International* 7, No. 19 October 1986

20 Greenfield, P. R. *Effective Prescribing* DHSS 1983

21 Benson, H. and Epstein, M. D. 'The Placebo Effect' *JAMA* 232 (12), 1975 pp. 1225–1227

22 Bell, J. S. *Applied Therapeutics 6* 1964

23 Braithwaite, A., Cooper, P. 'Study on the Effects of Tablet Colour in the Treatment of Anxiety State' *BMJ 282*, 1981 pp. 1576–1578

24 Adler, H. M., Hammett, V. O. 'The Doctor–Patient Relationship Revisited – An Analysis of the Placebo Effect' *Ann. of Int. Med 78*, 1973 pp. 595–598

25 Harris C. 'Prescribing – A Suitable Case for Treatment' Occasional Paper, RCGP 1985

4 The Tyranny of Excellence

1 Medawar, Sir Peter *The Hope of Progress* Methuen 1972

2 Needham, J. *The History of Scientific Thought* Cambridge University Press 1956

3 Elstein, A. *et al. An Analysis of Clinical Reasoning* Harvard 1978

4 Crombie, D. L. 'Diagnostic Process' *J. of the Royal College of General Practitioners 6*, 1963 pp. 579–589

5 Miller, D. (ed) *A Pocket Popper* Fontana 1983

6 Illich, I. *Limits to Medicine* Pelican 1977

7 *Alternative Therapy* British Medical Association Board of Education and Science 1986

8 *Physical Defects – The Pathway to Correction* American Child Health Association NY 1934 Ch. 8, pp. 80–96

9 Baum, M. 'Fashion v. Facts' *World Medicine* 2 April 1983 pp. 44–47

10 Reason, P., Rowan, J. (eds) *Human Inquiry* Wiley 1981

11 Metroff, I., Kilmann, R. *Methodological Approaches to Social Science* Josey Bass 1978

12 Corker, Professor J. Letter to the *Guardian* 20 May 1988

13 Metroff, I. *op. cit.*

14 Gillon, R. *Philosophical Medical Ethics* Wiley 1986 p. 70

15 *Ibid.*

16 Baum, M. *op. cit.*

17 Faulder, C. Quote from *Whose Body Is It?* Virago 1985 p. 83

18 HRH The Prince of Wales Presidential Address to the British Medical Association 14 Dec. 1982

5 The Planet Strikes Back

1 Ward, B., Dubos, R. *Only One Earth* Penguin 1972; Dubos, R. *Man, Medicine and Environment* Pall Mall Press 1968
2 Adams, F. *The Genuine Works of Hippocrates 1*, 1849 p. 190
3 Selye H. *The Stress of Life* McGraw-Hill 1978
4 Meadows, Donella H. *et al*. *Limits to Growth* Signet 1972
5 Ehrlich, P. *Population Bomb* Pan 1971
6 Ward B., Dubos R. *ibid*.
7 Melvyn Howe, G. *Man, Environmental Disease in Britain* David & Charles 1972
8 Bulton, J. *How to be Green* Century-Hutchinson 1989
9 Andur, M. O. Hazards to health: air pollution and human health – chronic biologic effects *New Engl. J. Med.* 266(11), 1962 pp. 555–556
10 McCormick, J. *The Users Guide to the Environment* Kogan Page 1985
11 Higgins, R. *The Seventh Enemy* Pan 1978; BMA *The Medical Effects of Nuclear War* Wiley 1983; Croall, S., Sempler, K. *Nuclear Power for Beginners* Writers & Readers 1985
12 McCormick, J. *The Users Guide to the Environment* Kogan Page 1985
13 McCormick, J. *op. cit*. Higgins, R. *op. cit*.
14 McCormick J. *op. cit*.
15 Higgins, R. *op. cit*.
16 *Ibid*.
17 Ballentine, R. *Diet and Nutrition* Himalayan Institute 1978
18 Bland, J. *Medical Application of Clinical Nutrition* Keats 1983
19 Hume Hall, R. *Food for Nought* Vintage 1976
20 Lewith, G.T. and Kenyon, J. *Clinical Ecology* Thorsons 1985
21 Hanssen, M. *E for Additives – the complete 'E' number guide* Thorsons 1985
22 Board, J., Board, C. *Sacred Waters* Granada 1985
23 Melvyn Howe, G. *op. cit*.

6 The Patient Wakes Up

1 Personal communication
2 Parsons, T. *The Social System* Routledge & Kegan Paul 1951
3 Johnson, T. 'The Professions in the Class Structure' in R. Scase (ed.), *Industrial Society Class Cleavage and Control* Allen & Unwin 1977 p. 106

4 Willis, E. *Medical Dominance – Division of Labour in Australian Health Care* Sydney Allen & Unwin 1983

5 *Complaints and Disorders – The Sexual Politics of Sickness* London Writers and Readers Publishing Co-operative 1976

6 Oppenheimer, M. 'The Proletarianization of the Profession' in Halmos, P. (ed.) *Professionalisation & Social Change* University of Keele 1973 pp. 213–228

7 Bennett, G. *Patients and their Doctors* Baillière-Tindall 1979

8 Boston Women's Health Collective Inc. *Our Bodies, Ourselves* NY Simon & Schuster 1975

9 Faulder, C. *Whose Body Is It?* Virago 1985

10 *Ibid.*

11 Gillon, R. *Philosophical Medical Ethics* Wiley 1985

12 *Handbook of Medical Ethics* British Medical Association 1984

13 *Ibid.*

14 *Ibid.*

15 *Ibid.*

16 *Professional Conduct and Discipline – Fitness to Practise* GMC 1985

17 Mumford, E. *Medical Sociology. Patients Providers and Policies* NY London House 1983

18 Revans, R. W. *The Morale and Effectiveness of General Hospitals* Oxford University Press 1964

19 *Project 2000: The New Preparation for Practice* UK Central Council for Nursing, Midwifery and Health Visiting 1986

20 *Neighbourhood Nursing: A Focus for Care* Report of the Community Nursing Review (Chairman: Julian Cumberledge), HMSO 1986

21 Batchelor, I. McFarlane, J. *Multi-disciplinary Clinical Teams* Based on the working papers of the Royal Commission on the NHS 1970 King's Fund Project Paper No. RC 12 1980

22 Marre, A. 'A Health Commissioner's View of Consumer Problems.' A paper from the Symposium on Inter-professional Learning. CETSW University of Nottingham 1979

23 Bligh, D. 'Some Principles for Inter-professional Learning and Teaching.' A paper from the Symposium on Inter-professional Learning. CETSW University of Nottingham 1979

24 Huntingdon, J. 'Factors Affecting Inter-professional Collaboration in Primary Health Care Settings.' Paper delivered

to the Royal Society of Medicine – Forum on Medical Communication 1987

25 Pietroni, P. C. Unpublished research conducted within a multi-disciplinary seminar in the undergraduate training of the Department of General Practice, St Mary's Hospital Medical School, Paddington 1988–1990

26 Griffiths, R. *Community Care: Agenda for Action* A report to the Secretary to State for Social Services HMSO 1988

7 The Planners Move In

1 Iliffe, S. *The NHS – A Picture of Health* Laurence & Wishart 1983

2 Newell, K. (ed.) *Health by the People* World Health Organisation 1975

3 Turner, B. *Medical Power and Social Knowledge* Sage 1987

4 Iliffe, S. *op. cit.*

5 *Report of the Royal Commission on Doctors' and Dentists' Remuneration* (Chairman: Sir Henry Pilkington) HMSO 1960

6 *Report of the Committee on Local Authority and Allied Personal Services* (Chairman: Lord Frederick Seebohm) HMSO 1968

7 *Report of the Committee on Senior Nursing Staff Structure* (Chairman: Brian Salmon) HMSO 1966

8 *Inequalities in Health Report* (Chairman: Sir Douglas Black) DHSS 1980

9 *Public Health in England Report* (Chairman: Sir Donald Acheson) HMSO 1988

10 Stowe, Sir K. *On Caring for the National Health* The Nuffield Provincial Hospitals Trust 1988

8 The Profession Reacts

1 *Report of the Committee of Inquiry into the Regulation of the Medical Profession* (Chairman: Sir Alexander Merrison) HMSO 1975

2 Porter, A. *et al.* 'Stress and the General Practitioner'. In Payne, R. L. & Firth-Cozens, J. F. (eds) *Stress in Health Professionals* Wiley 1987 pp. 45–69

3 Freudenberger, H. J. 'Staff Burn-Out' *Journal of Social Issues* *30* (1), 1980 pp. 159–165

4 Richards, C. *The Health of Doctors* King's Fund 1989

5 Murray, R. M. 'The Alcoholic Doctor' *British Journal of Hospital Medicine 17*, 1977 pp. 144–149

6 *Occupational Mortality* The Registrar General's decennial supplement 1970–72 HMSO 1978

7 Gerber, L. A. *Married to Their Careers* Tavistock 1983

8 Richards, C. *op. cit.*

9 Welner, A. *et al.* 'Psychiatric Disorders Among Professional Women *Archives of General Psychiatry 36*, 1979 pp. 169–173

10 *Neighbourhood Nursing: a Focus for Care* Report of the Community Nursing Review (Chairman: Julian Cumberledge), HMSO 1986

11 Rank, S. Jacobson, C. 'Hospital Nurses' Compliance with Medication Overdose Orders' *Journal of Health & Social Behaviour 9*, 1977 pp. 52–64

12 Eaton, G., Webb, B. 'Boundary Encroachment: Pharmacists in the Clinical Setting' *Sociology of Health & Illness 1*, 1979 pp. 69–89

13 *Alternative Therapy* British Medical Association Board of Education and Science 1986

14 Illich, I. *Limits to Medicine* Pelican 1977

15 de Kadt, E. *Inequality and Health* University of Sussex 1975

16 McKeown, I. *The Role of Medicine* Blackwell 1981

17 Kennedy, I. *The Unmasking of Medicine* Allen & Unwin 1981

18 White, E. *et al.* 'Ecology of Medical Care' *Eng. J. Med. 265*, 1961 pp. 885–892

19 Becker, H. *et al.* 'The Fate of Idealism in Medical Schools' *Am. Sociol. Rev. 23*, 1958 p. 50; 'Medical Students Medical Schools and Society During Three Eras' in Coombs, R. M., Vincent, C. E. (eds) *Psychological Aspects of Medical Training* Springfield, Ill. Charles C. Thomas 1971

20 Parlow, J., Robertson, A. 'Personality Traits of First Year Medical Students' *Brit. J. Med. Education 8*, 1974 pp. 8–12

21 Pietroni, P. C. *Review of Responses by Medical Students to Interviewing Course* St Mary's Hospital Medical School London 1986

22 Horder, J. *et al.* 'An Important Opportunity' *BMJ* 1984, 19 May pp. 1507–1511

9 The Feminine Principle

1 Lyons, A., Petrucelli, R. J. *Medicine, an Illustrated History* Abrams 1978
2 *Ibid*.
3 Cirlot, J. E. *A Dictionary of Symbols* Routledge & Kegan Paul 1962; Cooper, J. C. *An Illustrated Encyclopaedia of Traditional Symbols* Thames & Hudson 1982 p. 149
4 Martin, E. *The Women in the Body* Oxford University Press 1987
5 Laquer, T. *Female Orgasm Generation and the Politics of Reproductive Biology* 1986 pp. 35, 45
6 *Ibid*.
7 Martin, E. *op. cit*.
8 Ganong, W. *Review of Medical Physiology* 12 ed. Los Altos C. A. Lange 1983
9 Shorter, E. *A History of Women's Bodies* Pelican 1983 pp. 36, 42
10 *Ibid*.
11 *Ibid*.
12 Lewis, J. *The Politics of Motherhood* Croom Helm 1980 p. 126
13 Morris, N. 'Human Relations in Obstetrics' *Lancet* 23 April 1960 pp. 913–915
14 Arms, A. *Immaculate Deceptions* Houghton Mifflin 1975
15 Kitzinger, S. *The Experience of Childbirth* Gollancz 1962
16 Oakley, A. *The Captured Womb* Blackwell 1984
17 Savage, W. *A Savage Enquiry* Virago 1986
18 Palmer, G. *The Politics of Breastfeeding* Pandora 1988 p. 176
19 *Ibid*.
20 Lewin, E., Olesen, V. *Women, Health and Healing* Tavistock 1985
21 Orbach, S. *Fat is a Feminist Issue* Hamlyn 1979
22 Turner, B. *Medical Power and Social Knowledge* Sage 1987 p. 110
23 Roberts, H. *Patient Patients* Pandora Press 1985 p. 20
24 *Ibid*.
25 Ehrenreich, B., English, D. *Complaints & Disorders: The Sexual Politics of Sickness* London Writers & Readers Publishing Co-operative 1976

10 The Dignifying of Death

1 Evans, Wentz *The Tibetan Book of the Dead* Causeway Books 1973
2 *Report on a National Survey concerning Patients Nursed at Home* Marie Curie Memorial Foundation 1952
3 Hinton, J. 'Mental and Physical Distress in the Dying' *Quarterly Journal of Medicine* 32, 1963 pp. 2–21
4 Acring, C. D. *The Understanding Physician* Detroit Wayne State University Press 1971
5 Kübler-Ross, E. *On Death and Dying* Tavistock 1970
6 Hertz, R. *Death and the Right Hand* Cohen & West 1960
7 Rouse, W. H. D. (trans.) *The Great Dialogues of Plato* American Library pp. 461–521
8 Aries, P. *The Hour of Our Death* Penguin, 1983
9 Illich, I. *op. cit.*
10 Ramsey, P. *The Indignity of Death* Hastings Centre Study (2) 1974
11 Kübler-Ross, E. *op. cit.*
12 Cartwright, A., Hockey, L., Anderson, J. *Life Before Death* Routledge & Kegan Paul 1973
13 Saunders, C. *The Management of Terminal Malignant Disease* Edward Arnold 1984
14 Wilkes, E. *A Source Book of Terminal Care* Sheffield University Press 1985
15 Kelly, O. E. *Make Today Count* Delacorte Press 1975
16 Parkes, C. *Bereavement Studies of Grief in Adult Life* Tavistock Publications 1972
17 Parkes, C. 'Evaluation of a Bereavement Service' *Preventative Psychiatry* 1, 1981 p. 179

11 The Gentler Way with Cancer

1 Facts on Cancer. Cancer Research Campaign 1987
2 Hayward, J., Klugman, D. J. *et al.* 'Treatment of early breast cancer: a report after 10 years of a clinical trial' *Br. Med. J. 2*, 1972 pp. 423–429
3 Cassileth, B. R. 'The Social Implications of Questionable Cancer Therapies' *Cancer 63*, 1989 pp. 1247–1250
4 Pietroni, P. C. 'The Case for a Real Alternative in the Treatment of Cancer' in *Cancer Topics 6* (2), 1986 pp. 22–23

5 Fiore, N. 'Fighting Cancer – One Patient's Perspective *New Eng J Med 300*, 1979 pp. 284–289

6 Lerner, M., Remen, R. N. 'Varieties of Integral Cancer Therapies' *Advances 2* (3), 1985 pp. 14–33; Lerner, M. 'A Report on Complementary Cancer Therapies' *Advances 2* (1), 1985 pp. 31–43; Lerner, M. 'Tradecraft of the Commonweal Cancer Heal Program' *Advances 4* (3), 1987 pp. 11–25

7 *Ibid.*

8 Cassileth, B. R. 'Contemporary Unorthodox Treatments' *Am. Intern. Med.* 101, 1984 pp. 105–112

9 Cosh, J., Sikora, K. 'Conventional and Complementary Treatment for Cancer: Time to Join Forces' *BMJ 298*, 1989 pp. 1200–1201

10 Fiore, N. *op. cit.* 1979; Dreher, H. 'Cancer and Mind: Current Concepts in Psycho-Oncology Advances' *Advances 4* (3), 1987 pp. 27–43

11 Cassileth, B. R. 'After Laetrile, What?' *New Engl. J. Med.* 306, 1982 pp. 1482–1483; Cassileth, B. R. 1984 *op. cit.*

12 Cassileth, B. R. 1982 *op. cit.*; Cassileth, B. R. 1984 *op. cit.*; Lerner, M. 1987 *op. cit.*

13 Cassileth, B. R. 1982 *op. cit.*

14 Fiore, N. *op. cit.* 1979; Thomas, C. B. 'Cancer and the Youthful Mind: A Forty Year Perspective' *Advances 5* (2), 1988 pp. 42–58; Benson, M. 'The Placebo Effect: A Neglected Aspect in the Care of Patients' *JAMA*, pp. 225–227; Hunter, M. 'Unproven Dietary Methods of Treatment of Oncology Patients' *Recent Res. Cancer Res. 108*, 1988 pp. 235–238

15 Cassileth, B. R. 1982 *op. cit.*

16 Lerner, M., Remen, R. N. *op. cit.*

17 Holohan, T. V. 'The Medical Community and Unorthodox Therapy' *op. cit.*; Herbert, V. 'Unproven (Questionable) Dietary and Nutritional Methods in Cancer Prevention and Treatment' *Cancer 58*, 1986 pp. 1930–1941; *Subcommittee on Unorthodox Therapies, American Society of Clinical Oncology Ineffective Cancer Therapy: A Guide for the Layperson 1* (2), 1983 pp. 154–163; Danielson, K. J. *et al.* 'Unconventional Cancer Remedies' *J. Canadian Med. Assoc. 138*, 1988 pp. 1005–1011; Clinical Oncology Group 'New Zealand Cancer Patients and Alternative Medicine *NZ Med. J. 100*, 1987 pp. 100–103

18 Thomas, C. B. 'Family Attitudes Reported in Youth as Poten-

tial Predictors of Cancer' *Psychosom. Med. 41*, 1979 pp. 287–302

19 Shaffer, J. W. *et al.* 'Family Attitudes in Youth as a Possible Precursor of Cancer Among Physicians: A Search for Explanatory Mechanisms *J. Behav. Med.* 5 (2), 1982 pp. 143–163

20 Thomas C. B. 'Cancer and the Youthful Mind: A Forty Year Perspective' *loc. cit.*

21 Shaffer, J. W. *et al.*, *op. cit.*

22 Thomas, C. B. *op. cit.*

23 Shaffer, J. W. *et al.*, *op. cit.*

24 *Ibid.*

25 Thomas, C. B. *op. cit.*; Shaffer, J. W. *et al.*, *op. cit.*; Cassileth, B. R. 'Psychological Correlates of Survival in Advanced Malignant Disease' *NEJM 312*, 1985 pp. 1551–1555

26 Dreher, H. *op. cit.*; Shaffer, J. W. *et al.*, *op. cit.*

27 Dreher, H. *op. cit.*

28 Bridge, L. R. *et al.* 'Relaxation and Imagery in the Treatment of Breast Cancer' *BMJ 297*, 1988 pp. 1169–1172

29 Willett, W. C., MacMahon, B. 'Diet and Cancer – An Overview (Pt. 2)' *NEJM 310*, 1984 pp. 697–703

30 Dreher, H. *op. cit.*

31 *Ibid.*

32 Hunter, M. *op. cit.*

12 The Managing of Misery

1 Stafford-Clark, D. *Psychiatry Today* Pelican 1963

2 Zilboorg, G. *History of Medical Psychology* NY Norton 1940

3 *Ibid.*

4 Fry, J., Brooks, D., McColl, I. *NHS Data Book* MTP Press 1984

5 Goffman, E. *Asylums* Penguin 1966

6 Szasz, T. *Myth of Mental Illness* Paladin 1972

7 Laing, R. D. *The Divided Self* Tavistock 1960

8 Scheff, T. J. *Being Mentally Ill* Weidenfeld & Nicolson 1966

9 Rosenheim, D. 'On Being Sane in Insane Places' 79, *Science* 1973 pp. 250–258

10 Meyer A. *Commonsense Psychiatry: Fifty-two Selected Papers* ed. Lief, A. McGraw-Hill 1948

11 Brown, G. W., Harris, T. *Social Origins of Depression* Tavistock 1978

12 Rogers, C. *Client Centered Therapy* Constable 1951
13 Frank, J. *Persuasion and Healing* Schocken 1974
14 Tuax, *et al*. 'Therapist empathy, genuineness and warmth and patient therapeutive outcome' *J. Consult. Psychol. 30*, 1966 pp. 395–401

13 The Return of the Spirit

1 Plato *Dialogues*
2 Fry, A. *Safe Space* Dent 1987
3 Jung, C. J. *Collected Works 16*, 1982 p. 59
4 Sargant, W. *Battle for the Mind* Pan 1960
5 Balint, E., Norell, J. (eds) *Six Minutes for the Patient* Tavistock 1973
6 Balint, M. *The Basic Fault* Tavistock 1984
7 Montagu, A. *Touching* Perennial Library Harper and Row 1973
8 Hamnett, F. S. 'Studies in the Thyroid Apparatus' *Am. J. Physiology 56*, 1921 pp. 196–204
9 Rheingold, H. 'The Maternal Affectional System of Rhesus Monkeys' in *Maternal Behavior in Mammals* Wiley 1963, p. 260
10 *Alternative Therapy* British Medical Association Board of Education and Science 1986
11 *Ibid.*
12 Fulder, S. *The Handbook of Complementary Medicine* 2nd ed OUP 1988
13 Wordsworth, W. *Lines upon Tintern Abbey*
14 Isherwood, M. *The Root of the Matter* Gollancz 1954
15 Pelletier, K. *Mind as Healer, Mind as Slayer* Allen & Unwin 1978
16 Locke, Hornig-Rowan *Mind and Immunology* Institute for Advancement of Health 1985
17 Coward, R. *The Whole Truth* Faber & Faber 1989

14 Opting In and Opting Out

1 Fry, J. *Self-Care* A report by an independent Working Party 1973

2 Horder, J., Horder, G. 'Illness in General Practice' *The Practitioner* 1954 pp. 173, 177; White, K. L. *et al.* 'The Ecology of Medical Care' *New Eng. J. of Medicine 268*, 1961 p. 885

3 Jefferys, M. *et al.* 'The Consumption of Medicines in a Working Class Housing Estate' *Brit. J. of Social & Preventive Medicine 14*, 1960 p. 164

4 Fry, J., Brooks, D., McColl, I. *NHS Data Book* 1984

5 Elliott-Binns, C. P. 'Analysis of Lay Medicine' *J. of RCGP 23*, 1973 p. 255

6 Donaher, K. 'Self-Treatment and Consultation' Paper presented to the Annual Meeting of the Medical Sociology Group of the British Sociological Association York 1975

7 Elliott-Binns, C. P. *op. cit.*

8 Helman, C. *Culture Health and Illness* John Wright 1984

9 Elliott-Binns, C. P. *op. cit.*

10 Steinman, R., Traunstein, D. 'Redefining Deviance: the self-help challenge to the human services *J. of Applied Behavioural Science 12* (3), 1976 p. 347

11 Herzlich, C. *Health or Illness* Academic Press 1974

12 Williamson, J. and Donaher, K. *Self-care in Health* Croom Helm 1978

13 Graham, S. *Lectures in the Science of Human Health* Boston 1839

14 Boston Women's Collective *Our Bodies, Ourselves* Simon & Schuster 1975

15 Fulder, S. *Handbook of Complementary Medicine* 2nd ed. OUP 1988

16 Pietroni, P. C. 'Alternative Medicine 1987' *J. of the Royal Society of Arts* October 1988 pp. 791–801

17 Reilly, D. 'Young Doctors' View on Alternative Medicine' *BMJ 287*, 1983 pp. 337–339

18 Wharton, R. W., Lewith, G. 'Complementary Medicine and the General Practioner' *BMJ 292*, 1986 pp. 1498–1500

19 Fulder, S., Monro, R. *The Status of Complementary Medicine in the United Kingdom* Threshold Foundation 1981

20 'Magic or Medicine?' *Which?* August 1981

21 Fulder, S. *op. cit.*

22 Mori Poll *The Times* 13 November 1989

23 *Alternative Therapy* British Medical Association Board of Education and Science 1986

24 Watt, Sir J. (ed.) *Talking Health* Royal Society of Medicine 1988

15 The Seeds Begin to Sprout

1 Innes Pearse, H., Crocker, P., Crocker, L. *The Peckham Experiment* George Allen & Unwin 1943; Williamson, G. Scott, Innes Pearse, H. *Synthesis and Sanity* Collins 1965; Innes Pearse, H. *The Quality of Life* Scottish Academic Press 1989

2 Innes Pearse, H. 'Periodic Overhaul of the Uncomplaining' *J. of the Royal College of General Practitioners* 20, 1970 p. 146

3 Innes Pearse, H. 1989 *op. cit.*

4 Pietroni, P. C., McLean, J., Walton, N. G. 'A Self-Care Programme in General Practice – A Feasibility Study' Special Report in *The Practitioner 231*, 1987 pp. 1226–1230; McLean, J., Pietroni, P. C. *Self-Care – Who Does Best? Soc. Sci. Med.* 30(5) 1990 pp. 591–596

5 Information Leaflet (No. 1) Marylebone Centre Trust 1988

6 *Ibid.*

7 *Ibid.*

8 *Ibid.*

9 *Ibid.*

10 *Ibid.*

11 Tudor-Hart, J. 'Reactive and Proactive Care: A Crisis' *Brit. J. Gen. Prac.* vol. 40, 1990, pp. 4–9

12 Tudor-Hart, J. *A New Kind of Doctor* Merlin 1988

Organisations

Cancer

BACUP (British Association for Cancer United Patients and their Families)
121–123 Charterhouse Street
London EC1M 6AA   (tel: 071-608 1661)
Information and advice on all forms of treatment from a team of doctors

Bristol Cancer Help Centre
Grove House, Cornwallis Grove
Clifton, Bristol BS9 1SY   (tel: 0272 743216)

Cancer Research Campaign
2 Carlton House Terrace
London SW1Y 5AR   (tel: 071-930 8972)

Complementary medicine

Council for Complementary and Alternative Medicine
38 Mount Pleasant
London WC1X 0AP   (tel: 071-409 1440)
Will identify local practitioners in acupuncture, chiropractic, herbalism, homoeopathy and osteopathy

Research Council for Complementary Medicine
5th floor, 60 Great Ormond Street
London WC1N 3JF   (tel: 071-833 8897)
Sponsors and publishes research; education for research; information service on research

The following organisations publish members' registers, which are available on request; some may be seen in a public library

Council for Acupuncture
38 Mount Pleasant
London WC1X 0AP   (tel: 071-837 8026)
Incorporates the four major acupuncture associations

British Chiropractors' Association
10 Greycoat Place
London SW1P 1SB   (tel: 071-222 8866)

National Institute of Medical Herbalists Ltd
Hon. Gen. Sec.: Mrs Chacksfield, 9 Palace Gate
Exeter EX1 1JA   (tel: 0392 426022)

Faculty of Homoeopathy
Royal London Homoeopathic Hospital
Great Ormond Street
London WC1N 3HR   (tel: 071-837 3091 ×72)
Medically qualified homoeopaths

Society of Homoeopaths Ltd
2 Artizan Road,
Northampton NN1 4HU   (tel: 0604 21400)
Non-medically qualified homoeopaths

General Council and Register of Osteopaths
56 London Street
Reading RG1 4SQ   (tel: 0734 576585)

Counselling services

British Association for Counselling
37a Sheep Street
Rugby, Warks CV21 3BX   (tel: 0788 78328/9)
*Publishes a directory of counselling and psychotherapy
resources*

CRUSE
126 Sheen Road
Richmond, Surrey TW9 1UR   (tel: 081-940 4818)
Bereavement counselling

Tavistock Clinic
120 Belsize Lane
London NW3 5BA   (tel: 071-435 7111)
Family counselling service

Death and dying

CRUSE
126 Sheen Road
Richmond, Surrey TW9 1UR   (tel: 081-940 4818)
Advice on practical problems

Elisabeth Kübler-Ross Foundation
PO Box 212
London NW8 7NW   (tel: 071-837 9796)
Counselling, seminars, videos

Diet and nutrition

British Society for Nutritional Medicine
Information Officer: Dr Alan Stewart
5 Somerhill Road
Hove, E. Sussex BN3 1RP   (tel: 0273 722003)

Ecology

Ecology Party
10 Station Parade
Balham High Road
London SW12 9AZ   (tel: 081-673 0045)

Friends of the Earth
26–28 Underwood Street
London N1 7JQ   (tel: 071-490 1555)

Feminine issues

AIMS (Association for Improvements in the Maternity Services)
Goose Green Barn
Much Hoole, Preston PR4 4TD   (tel: 0772 615840)

Feminist Library and Information Centre
1st floor, Hungerford House
Victoria Embankment
London WC2N 6PA   (tel: 071-930 0715)

Holistic health centres

Glyncorrwg Health Centre
Waun Avenue
Glyncorrwg, Port Talbot
South Wales SA13 3DP

Marylebone Health Centre
St Marylebone Parish Church
17 Marylebone Road
London NW1 5LT

Holistic medicine

British Holistic Medical Association
179 Gloucester Place
London NW1 6DX   (tel: 071-262 5299)

Hospice movement

St Christopher's Hospice
51 Lawrie Park Road
Sydenham
London SE26 6DZ   (tel: 081-778 9252)
*Runs a hospice information service, and publishes a directory of
hospices in the UK and the Republic of Ireland*

Mental health

National Association for Mental Health (MIND)
22 Harley Street
London W1N 2ED   (tel: 071-637 0741)

Patients' rights

Action for Victims of Medical Accidents
1 London Road
Forest Hill
London SE23 3TP   (tel: 081-291 2793)

Association of Parents of Vaccine Damaged Children
2 Stour Street,
Shipston-on-Stour, Warks CV36 4AP   (tel: 0608 61595)

Patients' Association
18 Victoria Park Square
Bethnal Green, London E2 9PF   (tel: 081-981 5675 & 5695)

Self-help organisations

The following directories list organisations giving information and advice on specific conditions, e.g. motor neurone disease, arthritis etc.

Self-Help and the Patient. Patients' Association. 10th ed. 1986

Health Help 1987/88, compiled by Nancy Duin. Bedford Square Press/NCVO for Thames TV Help! Programme

The Self-Help Guide, by Sally Knight and Robert Gann. Chapman and Hall, 1988

Index